Aids to Clinical Pharmacology and Therapeutics

For Churchill Livingstone:

Publisher: Timothy Horne
Project Editor: Dilys Jones
Copy Editor: Linda Pica
Indexer: Jill Halliday
Sales Promotion Executive: Marion Pollock

Aids to Clinical Pharmacology and Therapeutics

John Rees MA MD FRCP
Consultant Physician, Guy's Hospital, London
Senior Lecturer, United Medical and Dental Schools of Guy's and
St Thomas's Hospitals, London

James Ritter MA DPhil FRCP
Professor of Clinical Pharmacology, United Medical and Dental
Schools of Guy's and St Thomas's Hospitals, London

Roy Spector MD PhD FRCP
Emeritus Professor of Applied Pharmacology, University of London
Honorary Consultant Physician, Guy's Hospital, London

THIRD EDITION

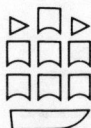

CHURCHILL LIVINGSTONE
EDINBURGH LONDON MADRID MELBOURNE NEW YORK AND TOKYO 1993

CHURCHILL LIVINGSTONE
Medical Division of Longman Group UK Limited

Distributed in the United States of America by
Churchill Livingstone Inc., 650 Avenue of the
Americas, New York, N.Y. 10011, and by
associated companies, branches and representatives
throughout the world.

First edition 1984
Second edition 1989
Third edition 1993

ISBN 0-443-04698-0

British Library Cataloguing in Publication Data
A catalogue record for this book is available from the British Library.

Library of Congress Cataloging in Publication Data
Rees, John, M.D., M.R.C.P.
    Aids to clinical pharmacology and therapeutics / John Rees, James
Ritter, Roy Spector. — 3rd ed.
        p.   cm.
    Rev. ed. of: Aids to clinical pharmacology and therapeutics /
Howard Rogers, Roy Spector. 2nd ed. 1989.
    Includes index.
    ISBN 0-443-04698-0
    1. Drugs—Handbooks, manual, etc.   2. Pharmacology—Handbooks,
manuals, etc.   3. Chemotherapy—Handbooks, manuals, etc.
I. Ritter, James. II. Spector, R. G. (Roy Geoffrey) III. Rogers,
Howard (Howard John) Aids to clinical pharmacology and therapeuti.
    [DNLM: 1. Drug Therapy—handbooks.   2. Pharmacology, Clinical—
—handbooks. QV 39 R328a]
RM301.12R44   1992
DNLM/DLC
for Library of Congress   92-49325

Produced by Longman Singapore Publishers Pte Ltd
Printed in Singapore

Contents

Preface

We all differ in our approach to learning in the medical course. In general, 'Aids' and 'Notes' have greater popularity with students than with their teachers. One possible explanation of this phenomenon is that such short-cut texts are academically poor and do not represent the real world because a practised doctor does not sieve through lists when confronted with a clinical problem. Students, on the other hand, gain confidence in seeing the imposition of some sort of order on the chaos of facts which confront them. Of course, in a subject such as clinical pharmacology, which is imperfectly understood in terms of mechanism and whose subject matter is in a constant state of flux, order may be spurious and illusory. Despite this, we have made an attempt to tame the facts and the material presented contains the nucleus of our courses at the United Medical Schools. Around this core is other material which may be of use for students taught elsewhere. Practice is geographically variable and a drug used widely in our hospital may be substituted by another in another institution. Therefore this book is in some respects overcomprehensive. Our advice is to use it in conjunction with a pen to emphasise the drugs and practices which are of importance in your hospital and medical course.

We believe this subject cannot be learnt in abstraction from a book but that the student should learn therapeutics at the bedside. The drug chart and the patient's response to each item on it should be sought with that eager attention with which you strain to hear an opening snap or pleural rub on your patients. In addition you should consult larger textbooks for discussion in depth of those aspects of particular relevance to the treatment of a difficult clinical problem. Of all the subjects in the medical curriculum, clinical pharmacology is the one which will be most widely applicable in your future career: the surgeon, psychiatrist or general practitioner requires just as sound a background in therapeutics as the cardiologist or gastroenterologist. All are users of drugs but all may also be abusers of drugs to the detriment of their patients. We hope that this little book may also assist qualified doctors reading for higher examinations or perhaps just reading. Students in other faculties such as pharmacy may also find some of the lists and tables a useful summary of the information required in their examinations.

London   H.J.R.
1989   R.G.S.

Acknowledgement

Howard Rogers, my previous co-author, died during the preparation of the second edition. My new collaborators John Rees and Jim Ritter have provided much new material in producing the third edition. They have rewritten large sections — in particular the cardiovascular and respiratory systems and the chapters on chemotherapy.

London   R.G.S.
1993

1. Drug absorption, distribution, metabolism and excretion

DRUG ABSORPTION

Transmembrane movement of drugs

Drugs must pass several membranes to reach site of action.

1. *Passive diffusion* — commonest and most important
   — non-ionised drug is lipid soluble and diffuses easily (so oil/water partition coefficient, pH and pK_a important).
2. *Active* — relatively unusual
   — drugs resembling natural substrate can be transported, e.g. methyldopa, levodopa, 5-fluorouracil, methotrexate uptake in gut; renal tubular secretion of weak acids and bases.
3. *Facilitated* — carrier-mediated but no energy required, e.g. B_{12}-intrinsic factor complex but not important for drugs.
4. *Pinocytosis* — physical engulfment by cell
   — little importance for drugs; vitamins A, D, E, K absorbed this way.

BIOAVAILABILITY

Relative amount of administered drug dose reaching systemic circulation and rate at which this occurs.

Different formulations can contain the same amount of drug but availability to body may be vastly different.

Bioequivalence — two or more pharmaceutical formulations produce comparable bioavailability characteristics in an individual when administered in equivalent dosage regimes.

Bioinequivalence — statistically significant difference in bioavailability between preparations.

Therapeutic inequivalence — clinically importance difference in bioavailability.

Absolute bioavailability — availability of a drug product relative to i.v. administration.

Relative bioavailability — availability as compared to recognised standard preparation.

Factors influencing bioavailability
1. Drug characteristics
   a. incomplete absorption
   b. first pass elimination.
2. Formulation characteristics
   a. compression and physical factors affecting formulation dissolution and solubility
   b. state of drug, e.g. surface area, particle size.
3. Interactions with other substances in gut — food, drugs.
4. Patient characteristics — disease (e.g. malabsorption, hepatic dysfunction)
   — gastrointestinal factors (motility, pH, blood flow)
   — genetic factors, e.g. acetylator status.

Bioavailability assessment
1. *Plasma data — single dose*
   a. time of peak plasma concentration
   b. peak plasma concentration
   c. area under plasma concentration, time curve (AUC).
   Usually oral and i.v. doses (D) given in random order to panel of subjects.

Since $(AUC)_{p.o.} = \dfrac{FD}{kV}$ & $(AUC)_{i.v.} = \dfrac{D}{kV}$

where F is bioavailability fraction if k and V remain constant between doses (k = elimination rate constant V = distribution volume)

$$F = \frac{(AUC)_{p.o.}}{(AUC)_{i.v.}}$$

   — *multiple dose*: as a, b, c above during a single dosage interval.
2. *Urine data*
   a. total fraction of dose excreted
   b. rate of drug excretion
   c. time of maximum excretion.
3. *Clinical observation and pharmacological effects*, e.g. salivary secretion, heart rate.

Potential for bioinequivalence of dosage forms

Low	Intermediate	High
Elixirs	Capsules	Compressed tablets
Syrups	Suspensions	Enteric-coated tablets
Solutions	Chewable tablets	Sustained release formulations
		Suppositories

Examples of drugs for which bioinequivalence demonstrated among marketed oral formulations:

Aspirin	Digoxin	Phenytoin
Chloramphenicol	Nitrofurantoin	Prednisolone
Chlordiazepoxide	Oxytetracycline	Warfarin

Therapeutic inequivalence shown in most of the above.
Bioinequivalence often results in therapeutic inequivalence if
therapeutic index low.

Sustained release preparations
Aim to prolong action of drugs with short $T_{1/2}$ by pharmaceutical
means, e.g. resin coated pellets in capsules, drug enclosed in wax or
plastic matrix.

Potential advantages
Prolonged effects
Improved compliance
Improved tolerability

May be valuable if:
1. short $T_{1/2}$ (1–8 h)
2. prolonged treatment necessary (improves compliance)
3. constant plasma levels needed for efficacy.

Potential disadvantages
1. Cost — more expensive than conventional tablets
2. Delayed absorption — delayed onset of action or failure of
   dissolution
   — increased first-pass effects
3. Prolonged toxicity
4. Increased risk of gut toxicity.

Enteric coated tablets or granules
Film coat (polymer like cellulose acetate phthalate) which resists
dissolution by stomach acid but disrupts or dissolves in alkaline
intestinal juice. Occasionally used to reduce gastric irritation, e.g.
aspirin, prednisolone.

FACTORS AFFECTING GASTROINTESTINAL DRUG ABSORPTION
1. Drug
   a. lipophilicity (e.g. oil/water partition coefficient)
   b. pKa
   c. metabolism in gut.
2. Formulation
Dissolution rate
3. Patient
   a. pH of gut
   b. rate of gastric emptying

    c. intestinal motility (transit time)
    d. surface area available for absorption
    e. presence of food in gut
    f. interactions with drugs in gut.

EFFECT OF FOOD ON DRUG ABSORPTION

Decreased absorption	Increased absorption
Tetracycline (milk, cottage cheese)	Propranolol
Methotrexate (milk)	Hydrochlorothiazide

ROUTES OF DRUG ADMINISTRATION

Sublingual/buccal absorption
1. Rapid absorption
2. Avoids first-pass gastrointestinal/hepatic elimination.
Examples: glyceryl trinitrate, oxytocin, methyltestosterone, buprenorphine.

Rectal administration
1. Only partially avoids first-pass metabolism.
2. Small surface area (passive absorption only) and drug may be expelled so absorption rate and bioavailability erratic.
3. Unsuitable for irritant drugs.
4. Drugs given as solution (retention enema) more rapid and efficient than given as solid formulation with wax base (suppository).
5. Useful if patient vomiting.
6. Used for systemic (e.g. theophylline, prochlorperazine, aspirin, oxycodone, indomethacin) or local (e.g. corticosteroids for inflammatory bowel disease) effects.

Intramuscular injection
1. Gastrointestinal and hepatic first-pass elimination avoided.
2. Absorption influenced by:
    a. local blood flow, massage and movement (e.g. exercise increases absorption; morphine absorption decreased after myocardial infarct; insulin absorption increased by sauna)
    b. site, e.g. lignocaine absorption absorbed faster from deltoid than vastus lateralis or gluteus maximus
    c. physical properties of drug — poorly water soluble drugs, e.g. diazepam, phenytoin precipitate in muscle and are poorly and erratically absorbed
    d. sex of patient — females may absorb less from gluteal injection.
Thus absorption less realiable than i.v. but solubility of drug not necessary.
3. Compliance ensured.

4. Onset of action more rapid than oral route.
5. Prolonged absorption can be produced by modification of injection
   — high viscosity vehicles like glycerin
   — fatty acid esters which slowly hydrolyse, e.g. fluphenazine
   decanoate for maintenance therapy in schizophrenia
   — water insoluble suspensions, e.g. procaine penicillin.
6. Complications
   a. pain, e.g. benzylpenicillin (maximum volume by i.m. is 4–5 ml)
   b. muscle and skin necrosis, e.g. digoxin, sterile or septic
      abscesses, pigmentation, e.g. iron
   c. sciatic nerve damage following gluteal injection
   d. elevated CPK may confuse diagnosis of myocardial infarction
   e. inadvertant intravascular injection.

Intravenous injection
1. Only route (apart from intra-arterial) when bioavailability
   considerations immaterial. Useful if:
   a. drug not absorbed p.o., e.g. gentamicin
   b. high first-pass elimination, e.g. lignocaine
   c. too irritant for i.m. or p.o. route, e.g. nitrogen mustard.
2. Almost instantaneous response but bolus of highly concentrated
   drug may cause cardiac, respiratory etc complications so i.v.
   injections should usually be slow.
3. Rate of administration flexible, e.g. nitroprusside, lignocaine, and
   plasma levels can be accurately maintained.
4. Drug administered may not be recalled c.f. p.o. when absorption
   can be reduced.
5. Only water-soluble or aqueous miscible systems can be given.
6. Tonicity of solution and lack of irritant properties important, some
   preparations cause thrombophlebitis, e.g. diazepam.
7. Risks
   a. anaphylaxis — greater with this route than others
   b. infection especially in immunosuppressed and seriously ill
   c. tissue damage if irritant drug extravasates, e.g. doxorubicin,
      actinomycin D, thiopentone.

Subcutaneous injection
1. Absorption influenced by same factors as i.m. injection but
   absorption slower and more erratic. Can sometimes increase
   bioavailability with hyaluronidase, local heat, massage, exercise.
2. Sustained release effect obtained from pellets of solid drug, e.g.
   testosterone replacement. Duration of insulin action controlled by
   crystalline size, e.g. semilente, lente, ultralente insulins.
3. Some injections painful, may cause necrosis or abscesses.

Percutaneous absorption
1. Drug absorption increased

    a. polythene occlusion increases skin hydration
    b. lipid solubility, e.g. poisoning by absorption of nicotine, organic phosphates through skin
    c. loss of stratum corneum
    d. site — plantar < scalp < posterior auricular
    e. age — steroids absorbed more readily in children than adults
    f. vehicle.
2. Topical application minimises systemic absorption — but can occur, e.g. steroids.
3. Route can be utilised to avoid first-pass elimination and prolong systemic action, e.g. glyceryl trinitrate.

Pulmonary absorption
1. Almost instantaneous absorption (large surface area).
2. Difficult to deliver drug into lung and to dose accurately — particles >10 μm impact in pharynx and nose and are swallowed. Optimum size is 1–2 μm which may reach alveoli and terminal bronchiole. Tidal volume and bronchial anatomy also important.
3. For local therapy, e.g. sodium cromoglycate, dexamethasone, isoprenaline but can use for systemic effects, e.g. ergotamine.
4. Anaesthetics.

DRUG DISTRIBUTION

Protein binding of drugs
Drugs can bind to tissue proteins but plasma protein binding best understood.
1. *Characteristics of binding*
    Usually reversible.
    Competition for binding may occur between drugs or drugs and endogenous compounds.
2. *Proteins responsible for binding*
    a. albumin — affinity for acidic drugs
                — 2 sites: I (warfarin site) also binds frusemide, phenytoin, valproate, indomethacin, glibenclamide, bilirubin.
                     II (diazepam site) also binds probenecid, salicylate, glibenclamide
                — fatty acids bind at separate site but can cause conformational change so altering drug binding
    b. α_1 acid glycoprotein — affinity for basic drugs, e.g. propranolol, imipramine, chlorpromazine, lignocaine
                             — protein increases with ESR so binding changes with inflammation
    c. α_1 globulin: steroids (transcortin)
                    vitamin B_{12}
                    thyroxine

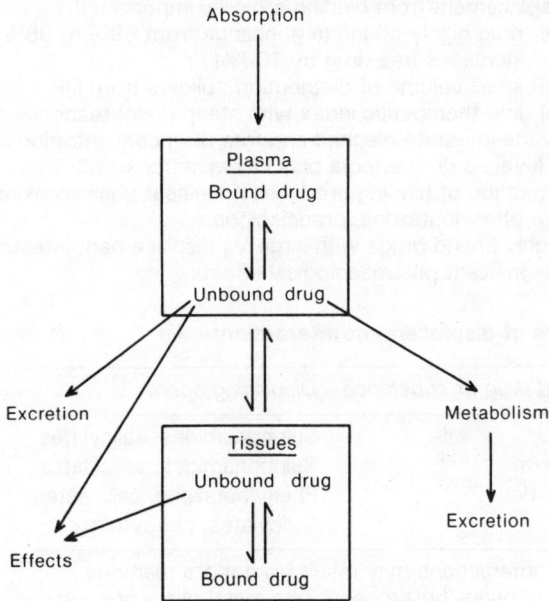

Absorption

Plasma
Bound drug

Unbound drug

Excretion

Tissues
Unbound drug

Metabolism

Excretion

Effects

Bound drug

Fig. 1.1

    d. α_2 globulin: copper (caeruloplasmin)
    e. β_1 globulin: iron (transferrin)
    f. lipoproteins, e.g. quinidine, imipramine
    g. erythrocytes, e.g. quinidine, propranolol
    h. tissue proteins, e.g. digitalis to Na^+, K^+, ATPase, vinca
       alkaloids to tubulin.
NB Not all drugs bound, e.g. heparin, allopurinol, isoniazid.

3. *Consequences of binding*
    a. drug transport within body
    b. drug reservoir if binding high
    c. only unbound ('free') drug may be available for action or
       metabolism so reduced binding may increase toxicity and
       clearance.
       Renal excretion: only unbound drug filtered at glomerulus so
       increased binding prolongs $T\frac{1}{2}$.
       Hepatic excretion: depends if drug has flow-dependent hepatic
       metabolism (e.g. propranolol) when increased binding delivers
       more drug or flow-independent (e.g. warfarin) where only
       unbound drug is eliminated
    d. bound drug cannot diffuse into tissues so binding determines
       volume of distribution and penetration into tissues, e.g. CSF,
       and secretions, e.g. saliva

e. displacement from binding clinically important if:
  (i) drug highly bound (e.g. change from 99% to 98% binding
       increases free drug by 100%)
  (ii) small volume of distribution (follows from (i))
  (iii) low therapeutic index with steep dose–response curve
BUT new steady-state reached and free drug concentration reaches
previous level so drug effects only increase transiently.
f. saturation of binding produces non-linear pharmacokinetics,
   e.g. phenylbutazone, prednisolone.
NB for highly bound drugs with large V_d displacement interactions
have no significant pharmacological effects.

Examples of displacement interactions

Displaced drug or substance	Displacing agent
Bilirubin	Sulphonamides, salicylates
Methotrexate	Sulphonamides, salicylates
Tolbutamide	Phenylbutazone, salicylates
Warfarin	Salicylates, phenytoin

NB some interactions may result from more than one
action, e.g. phenylbutazone inhibits metabolism of most
active (S–) isomer of warfarin.

DRUG METABOLISM

Drug metabolism chemically modifies drugs and may:
1. Abolish the activity (e.g. oxidation of barbiturates, phenytoin,
   alcohol; hydrolysis of suxamethonium, acetylcholine; conjugation
   of isoprenaline, salicylate).
or
2. Promote or increase activity (e.g. conversion of chloral to
   trichlorethanol, conversion of phenacetin to paracetamol; activation
   of cyclophosphamide to alkylating metabolites).
or
3. Produce no change in activity (e.g. dealkylation of tricylic antidepressants, benzodiazepines).
   Metabolism usually produces a more polar molecule which
increases drug elimination since it is less susceptible to tubular
reabsorption or active uptake in renal tubules or biliary system. Two
phases of metabolism:
Phase I — Metabolic modification (e.g. oxidation, reduction,
            hydrolysis)
Phase II — Synthesis — i.e. conjugation (e.g. with glucuronic acid,
            glycine, glutamine, sulphate, acetate)

	Phase I oxidising etc.		Phase II conjugating	
Drug	→	metabolites	→	conjugated metabolites
	enzymes		enzymes	

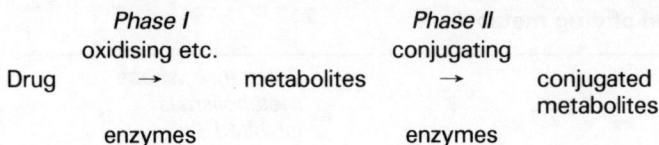

PHASE I METABOLISM

Occurs in 3 areas of cell:
1. smooth endoplasmic reticulum, e.g. barbiturates, pethidine
2. cytosol, e.g. ethanol, chloral
3. mitochondria, e.g. oxidation of tyramine by MAO.
   May also occur in plasma, e.g. succinylcholine hydrolysis by plasma pseudocholinesterase.
   Not all drugs broken down by enzymes, e.g. melphalan undergoes spontaneous hydroxylation to inactive metabolites.

PHASE II METABOLISM

Conjugation with:
1. glucuronic acid, e.g. salicylate, chloramphenicol, morphine
2. acetate, e.g. isoniazid, hydralazine, dapsone.

ENZYME INDUCTION

Enhancement of enzyme activity due to increase in the amount of enzyme protein present in the cell. Induction of enzymes concerned with drug metabolism usually accelerates destruction of drugs and reduces their action.
   Not only enzyme content of liver increased but organ size and blood flow also enhanced.
   Non-microsomal metabolism is not inducible.

Three groups of inducing agents
1. Substances which stimulate metabolism in many pathways, e.g. barbiturates, carbamazepine, rifampicin.
2. Polycyclic hydrocarbons (e.g. 3-methyl cholanthrene; 3-4 benzo-(a) pyrine) produce limited metabolic stimulation.
3. Steroids: mainly microsomal enzyme stimulation.

Smoking accelerates the metabolism of:
   amitriptyline
   pentazocine
   dextropropoxyphene.

Inhibition of drug metabolism

Drug	Substance whose metabolism is inhibited
Isoniazid	Phenytoin
Chloramphenicol	Phenytoin, tolbutamide
Ethanol (single large dose)	Chloral, tolbutamide, phenytoin, warfarin
Sulphonylureas	
Metronidazole	Acetaldehyde (from ethanol)
Procarbazine	
Cimetidine	Diazepam, ethanol, warfarin, propranolol, phenytoin

Metabolism by gut flora
Flora is a mixture of aerobic and anaerobic organisms.
   Microbial breakdown of hepatic conjugates frequently essential part of enterohepatic circulation.

Metabolism by gut mucosa
Mainly conjugations rather than Phase I metabolism in mucosal cells.
   Probably important for morphine, pentazocine, isoprenaline, tyramine, levodopa, oestrogens, progestogens, pivampicillin, flurazepam.
   Enzymes may be inhibited, e.g. MAOIs.

DRUG ELIMINATION

1. Metabolism (see above).
2. Storage — higher lipid soluble drugs in fat (e.g. DDT), heavy metals in bone, colloids in reticulo-endothelial system.
3. Excretion
   a. milk, sweat, tears, saliva. Usually quantitatively minor routes but may be of importance for toxicity, e.g. for baby in milk (dapsone, phenobarbitone, lithium)
   or
   can be used for therapeutic advantage, e.g. rifampicin for nasal carriage of meningococci; metronidazole in ulcerative gingivitis
   b. bile — secretion depends on structure, polarity, MW (? needs to be <325 in man)
      — carrier mediated active transport
      — competition within each compound class but not between classes

e.g. organic anions: penicillin, bile acids, bromsulphthalein
organic cations: tubocurarine, procainamide
unionised molecules: cardiac glycosides
— some drugs excreted unchanged in bile, e.g. rifampicin, adriamycin, erythromycin, others as conjugates, e.g. indomethacin, oestradiol, morphine, carbenoxolone

c. renal — often most important route of elimination of parent drug and/or metabolites if water-soluble and low MW < 500.

Three mechanisms:
1. Glomerular filtration — small molecules (<500 MW) so tightly protein bound not filtered.
2. Active tubular secretion — active carrier-mediated (requires energy, shows competition and saturation effects). 2 systems:
   a. Weak acids, e.g. acetazolamide, nitrofurantoin, penicillins, probenecid, phenobarbitone, salicylic acid, sulphathiazole
   b. Weak bases, e.g. amphetamine, chloroquine, imipramine, quinine.
3. Tubular reabsorption — may be active or passive
   — reabsorption governed by pH of tubular fluid and pK_a of drug
   — acids best eliminated in alkaline urine; bases best in acid urine.

For weak acids:

$$\frac{\text{Conc in urine}}{\text{Conc in plasma}} = \frac{1 + 10(\text{pH}_{urine} - pK_a)}{1 + 10(\text{pH}_{plasma} - pK_a)}$$

For weak bases:

$$\frac{\text{Conc in urine}}{\text{Conc in plasma}} = \frac{1 + 10(pK_a - \text{pH}_{urine})}{1 + 10(pK_a - \text{pH}_{plasma})}$$

Renal clearance (CL$_R$)

$$CL_R = \frac{dAe/dt}{C}$$

where dAe/dt is rate of excretion of drug in urine and C is plasma drug concentration. In practice it is found from UV/P where
U = concentration of drug excreted over a short period (say 1 hour);
V = volume of urine produced in that period; P = plasma conc at mid-point of time period.

If CL$_R$ > GFR tubular secretion must occur.
If CL$_R$ < GFR tubular reabsorption must occur.

But both processes may occur and obscure this simple pattern.

ENTEROHEPATIC CIRCULATION

Examples: thyroxine, oestrogens, stilboestrol, rifampicin, sulindac.

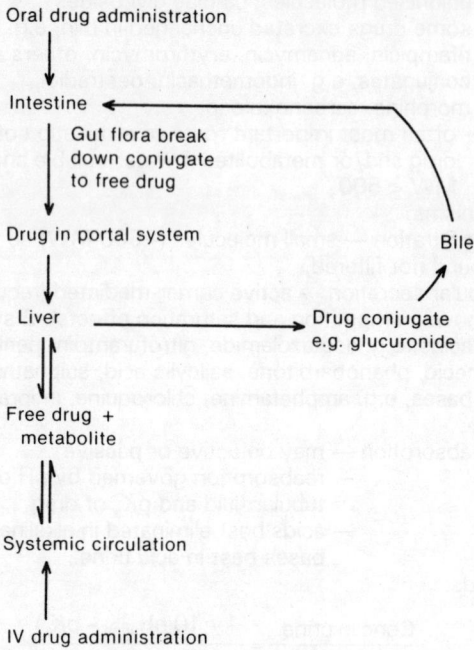

Oral drug administration

Intestine

Gut flora break
down conjugate
to free drug

Drug in portal system

Bile

Liver → Drug conjugate
e.g. glucuronide

Free drug +
metabolite

Systemic circulation

IV drug administration

Fig. 1.2

2. Other aspects of pharmacokinetics

Definition of pharmacokinetics
Study of the time course of drug absorption, distribution, metabolism and excretion (ADME) and of the mathematical relationships required in modelling this data.

Aims
To understand ADME processes and predict changes.
  These aims are possible since plasma drug concentration often correlates better with pharmacological response than does dose.

Compartment concept
In reality the body is composed of large number of compartments, e.g. each cell, but it is possible to lump together organs and tissues into larger compartments having no anatomical or physiological counterpart. The simplest pharmacokinetic model considers the body as 'black box' or single homogeneous compartment the volume of which determines the plasma concentration resulting from total amount of drug in the body. This *apparent volume of distribution* V is defined as

$$V = \frac{A}{C}$$

where A = amount of drug in body,
      C = plasma drug concentration
i.e.   A = VC   (1)
so that V is a proportionality factor relating dose to concentration.

V — has no physiological or anatomical meaning
  — seldom corresponds to anatomical body spaces
  — may exceed total body volume if drug concentrates in some region, e.g. fat.
C varies with time as drug undergoes ADME.

  Many drugs eliminated by *first-order kinetics*. This implies: rate of process ∝ amount of drug present. Called *linear kinetics*.

so
$$-\frac{dA}{dt} \propto A$$

(minus because amount of drug decreases with time)

so
$$\frac{dA}{dt} = -kA$$

and
$$\frac{dC}{dt} = -kC \text{ (since } C = A/V) \tag{2}$$

k is the first order elimination rate constant (units $[\text{time}]^{-1}$ e.g. h^{-1}, min^{-1}). Integrating from $t = 0$ where a dose of $A_{(0)}$ is given produces

$$A = A_{(0)}e^{-kt}$$

and
$$C = C_{(0)}e^{-kt} \tag{3}$$

Thus after a rapid (bolus) i.v. injection the plasma concentration, time curve is exponential for first order elimination:

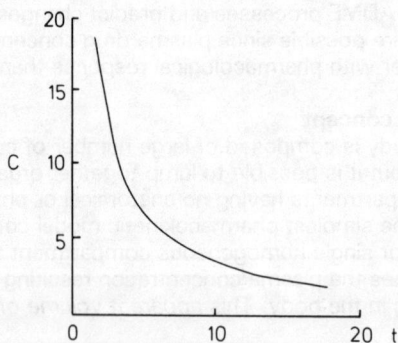

Fig. 2.1

This may be converted to a straight-line plot (easier to handle mathematically) by plotting

$$\log C = \log C_{(0)} - \frac{kt}{2.303}$$

i.e. ordinate intercept at $t = 0$ is $C_{(0)}$ (Fig. 2.2)

$$V = \frac{\text{Dose}}{C_{(0)}} \tag{4}$$

but this is of limited practical use for finding V since an i.v. drug injection is required.

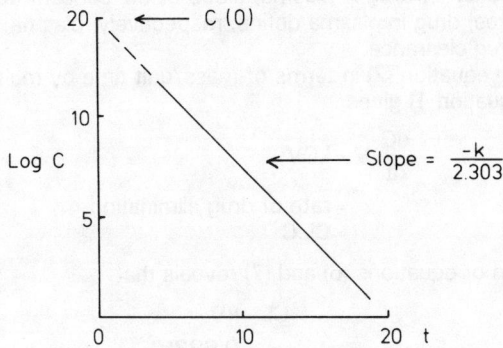

Fig. 2.2

More useful is to integrate equation (3) from t = 0 to ∞ which gives the area under the plasma concentration, time curve (AUC)

$$AUC = \int_0^\infty C_{(0)}e^{-kt}$$
$$= \frac{C_{(0)}}{k}$$

which can be substituted for $C_{(0)}$ in equation 4 to give

$$V = \frac{Dose}{k(AUC)} \tag{5}$$

AUC is found from direct measurement, e.g. planimeter, weighing cut-out curve, or by mathematical methods, e.g. trapezoidal rule.

Elimination half-life (T½)
Commonly used indicator of rapidity of drug elimination is time for any drug concentration to fall by half, i.e. has units of time (e.g. h, min).

As log C versus t plot is linear, $T½$ is same over entire time period

$$T½ = \frac{\log_e 2}{k} = \frac{0.693}{k} \tag{6}$$

Elimination clearance
As descriptors of drug elimination rate $T½$ and k are unsuitable because they also depend upon V. Clearance does not have this deficit.

Definition
Volume of biological fluid cleared of drug in unit time

$$CL = \frac{Rate\ of\ elimination}{Concentration}$$

Concentration of drug in plasma, blood or the concentration of unbound (free) drug in plasma define, respectively, plasma, blood or unbound drug clearance.

Rewriting equation (2) in terms of mass/unit time by multiplying by V (using equation 1) gives

$$-\frac{dC}{dt} \cdot V = kCV \qquad (7)$$

$$= \text{rate of drug elimination}$$
$$= CL.C \qquad (8)$$

Comparison of equations (6) and (7) reveals that

$$CL = kV$$
$$= \frac{0.693V}{T\tfrac{1}{2}}$$

Substituting for kV in equation (5) gives

$$CL = \frac{\text{Dose}}{\text{(AUC)}}$$

It is a physiologically meaningful parameter with units of flow (e.g. ml/min).

Total body clearance = sum of clearances by each eliminating organ (e.g. liver, kidneys).

NB
$$T\tfrac{1}{2} = \frac{0.693V}{CL}$$

so drug $T\tfrac{1}{2}$ can be long either because CL is low or V is large.

First pass effects

Drugs with high hepatic extraction ratios tend to have high first-pass (or pre-systemic) elimination after oral absorption, i.e. large proportion of drug is eliminated by the liver before it reaches general circulation.

Hepatic first-pass metabolism explains why despite complete absorption from the gut a drug may be much less effective than after i.v. dosing.

First-pass effects also occur due to intestinal mucosal metabolism (after oral administration), e.g. isoprenaline, chlorpromazine, and pulmonary metabolism (after aerosol inhalation), e.g. isoprenaline, nicotine.

Extent of first-pass elimination is predictable since

$$E = \frac{CL_H}{Q_H}$$

and the fraction of an orally administered drug reaching the systemic circulation

$$f_0 = 1 - E$$

Drugs with high hepatic first-pass elimination include propranolol, glyceryl trinitrate, pethidine, dextropropoxyphene.

Two-compartment models may be needed to explain the biphasic fall in log plasma concentration seen after i.v. drug injection:

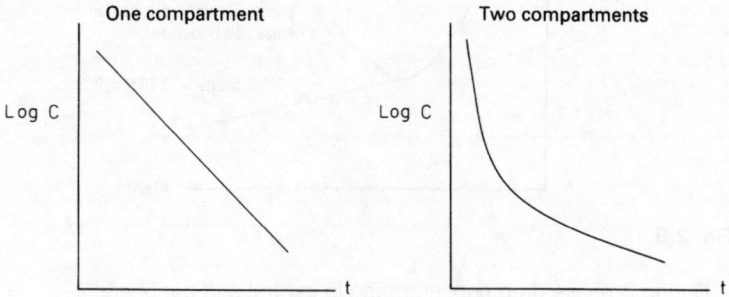

Fig. 2.3

The model involves a central compartment and a more slowly equilibrating deep or peripheral compartment.

Movement between compartments is by first order processes characterised by microconstants k_{12}, k_{21}.

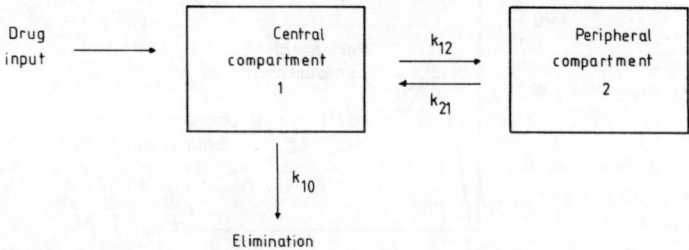

Fig. 2.4

The plasma concentration, time profile is described by

$$C = Ae^{-\alpha t} + Be^{-\beta t}$$

A, B, α and β can be obtained from the plasma concentration, time curve

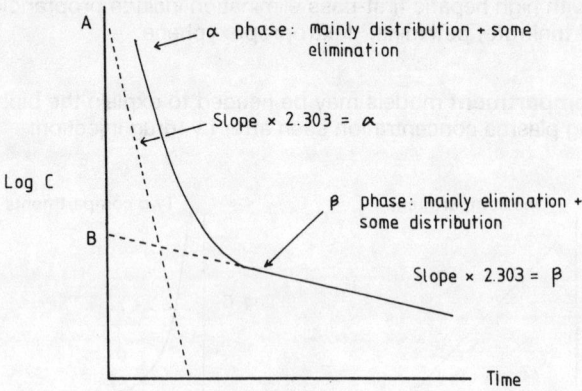

Fig. 2.5

During β-phase drug concentration in central and peripheral compartment declines in parallel (i.e. kinetic homogeneity attained). Plasma monitoring samples are best taken during this phase.

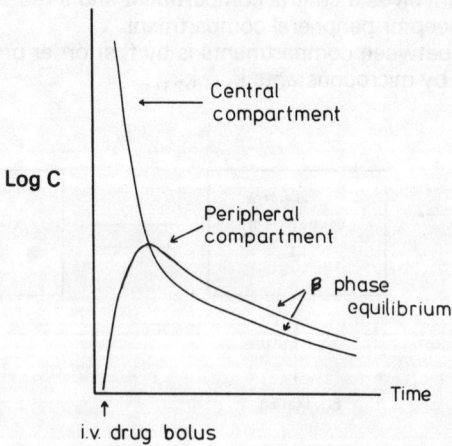

Fig. 2.6

$$\text{Distribution half life} = T_{\frac{1}{2}\alpha} = \frac{0.693}{\alpha}$$

$$\text{Disposition half life} = T_{\frac{1}{2}\beta} = \frac{0.693}{\beta}$$

If unspecified, $T_{1/2\beta}$ is 'half-life' for a 2-compartment drug.

Consequences of first order (linear) kinetics
1. $T_{1/2}$ is constant.
2. AUC $\propto$ dose.
3. Composition of drug products excreted independent of dose.
4. Amount of drug excreted unchanged in urine $\propto$ dose.
5. $C_{ss} \propto$ dose.

Saturation or zero order kinetics
In some cases the rate of elimination processes may not be proportional to drug amount or concentration. Many elimination processes occur via enzymes or carrier mediated systems which for some drugs become saturated in the therapeutic dose or concentration range.

This results in
1. Non-linear elimination kinetics:

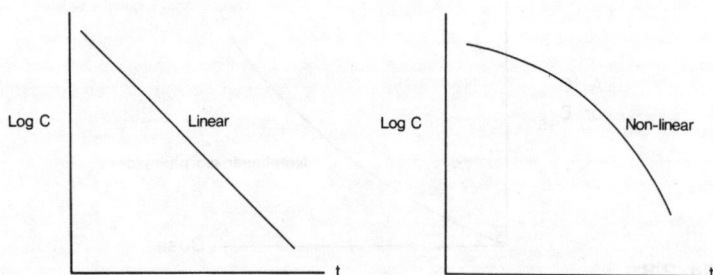

Fig. 2.7

2. $T_{1/2}$ increases with dose.
3. AUC is not proportional to amount of available drug — as a corollary steady state plasma concentration is not directly proportional to dose: see Fig. 2.8.
4. Saturation of capacity-limited processes may be affected by other drugs requiring same process, i.e. drug interactions common.
5. Composition of drug metabolites may vary with dose as one pathway becomes saturated and drug 'spills-over' into another pathway with higher capacity but lower affinity.
6. Amount of unchanged drug excreted in urine not proportional to dose.

Elimination described by Michaelis-Menten equation

$$\text{Elimination rate} = \frac{dC}{dt} = -\frac{V_{max}C}{K_m + C}$$

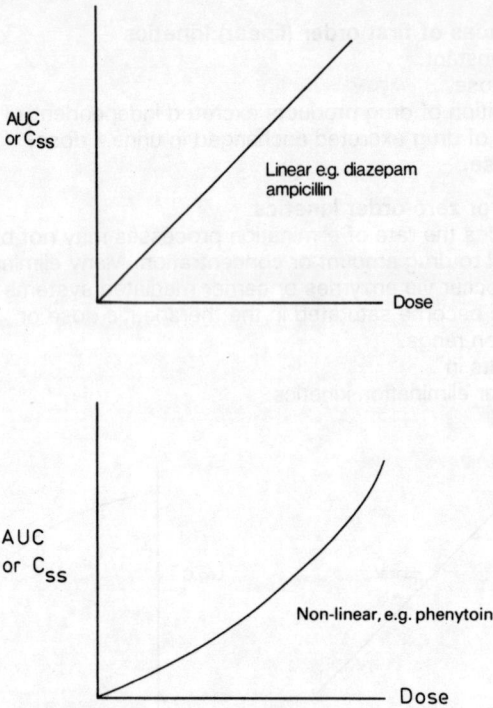

Fig. 2.8

where V_{max} = maximum velocity of process,
K_m = Michaelis constant = velocity at $V_{max}/2$

Non-linear kinetics
If $K_m \gg C$

$$\frac{dC}{dt} = \frac{-V_{max}C}{K_m}$$

$$= \text{constant} \times C$$

i.e. first-order kinetics are an extreme case of Michaelis-Menten kinetics. Also if $K_m \ll C$

$$\frac{dC}{dt} = -V_{max}$$

$$= \text{constant}$$

This is zero order kinetics, i.e. rate of process is independent of drug concentration.

Drugs exhibiting non-linear kinetics include:
ethanol; phenytoin; aspirin and salicylates; prednisolone; dicoumarol;
theophylline (?); chloroquine (?); overdoses with barbiturates and
tricyclic antidepressants (?); 5-fluorouracil; vincristine.

Non-linear kinetics important because:
1. Modest changes in drug dose may produce unexpected toxicity.
2. Elimination of drug and attainment of steady state takes
   unexpectedly long.
3. Changes in drug availability, e.g. changing formulation, can produce
   adverse effects.
4. May be more liable to competitive drug–drug interactions.

Multiple dosing
When drug is given in multiple doses if dose interval (τ) is small
relative to $T_{1/2}$, drug accumulates in the body until a steady state is
achieved when amount of drug given in dose interval = amount of
drug eliminated in dose interval. The time to attain steady state is
roughly 5 half-lives.
   A loading dose L can be given to achieve steady state more rapidly

$$L = \frac{\text{Maintenance dose } (A_{(0)})}{1 - e^{-kt}}$$

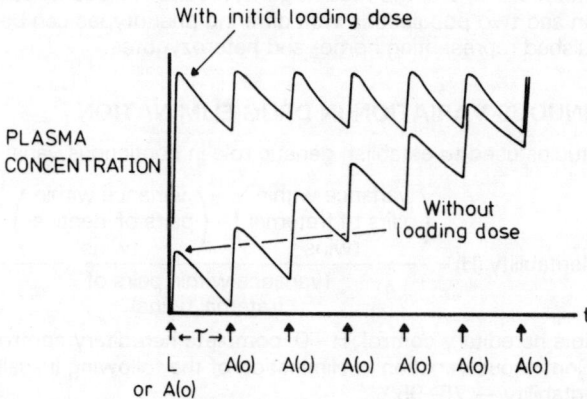

Fig. 2.9

3. Pharmacogenetics

Genetic influences mainly affect:
  drug metabolism
  responsiveness to drugs
but can also affect:
  absorption
  protein binding
  volume of distribution
  excretion
although these aspects less studied.

Polygenic effects produce continuous variation; *genetic polymorphism* (often the result of a single mutant gene) results in discontinuous variation and two populations with differing phenotypes can be distinguished representing homo- and heterozygotes.

CONTINUOUS VARIATION IN DRUG ELIMINATION

Twin studies used to establish genetic role in continuous variation:

$$\text{Heritability (H)} = \frac{\left(\begin{array}{c}\text{variance within}\\ \text{pairs of fraternal}\\ \text{twins}\end{array}\right) - \left(\begin{array}{c}\text{variance within}\\ \text{pairs of identical}\\ \text{twins}\end{array}\right)}{\left(\begin{array}{c}\text{variance within pairs of}\\ \text{fraternal twins}\end{array}\right)}$$

(Negligible hereditary control, H = 0; complete hereditary control, H = 1) Continuous variation in elimination of the following (usually with high heritability — 75–95%):

alcohol   chlorpromazine   warfarin
aspirin   imipramine   phenytoin

CONTINUOUS VARIATION IN PROTEIN BINDING
e.g. warfarin

	Heritability Index
Warfarin-albumin association constant	0.89
Number of drug binding sites/albumin molecule	0.85

DISCONTINUOUS VARIATION IN DRUG METABOLISM
Acetylation polymorphism
Due mainly to difference in activity and amount of hepatic
N-acetyltransferase; several primary amine drugs show bimodal
acetylation in man. Classically populations termed fast and slow
acetylators because $T\frac{1}{2}$ isoniazid is 50–100 minutes in former and
100–250 minutes in latter. Some drugs, e.g. dapsone, have same $T\frac{1}{2}$
in both phenotypes but ratio of acetylated metabolite to parent
compound greater in fast acetylators.

Inheritance. Rapid acetylation is autosomal dominant.

Prevalence

Ethnic group	% Rapid acetylators
Canadian eskimos	100
Japanese	88
Britons	38
Egyptians	18

Clinical relevance

Drug	Phenotype	Clinical effect
Isoniazid	Slow	Develop SLE more frequently. Peripheral neuropathy commoner. More prone to phenytoin toxicity if given isoniazid.
	Fast	?More prone to isoniazid hepatitis. ?Less rapid control of TB on once weekly isoniazid regimes.
Procainamide	Slow	Develop antinuclear antibodies and SLE more frequently.
Hydralazine	Slow	Develop antinuclear antibodies and SLE more frequently (but HLA-Dw4 more highly correlated).
	Fast	?Require higher doses to control hypertension.

Other drugs showing acetylation polymorphism are sulphadimidine,
aminoglutethimide and amino metabolites of nitrazepam and
clonazepam.

Some evidence that slow acetylators more likely to develop 'spontaneous' SLE and diabetic peripheral neuropathy.

Polymorphism of oxidation phenotype

Few isolated pedigrees (p-oxidation of phenytoin; O-de-ethylation of phenacetin) reported. Recent intensive investigation of two systems:

a. *Oxidation of debrisoquine*. Based on 0–8 h urine following 10 mg dose p.o.:

$$\text{Metabolic ratio} = \frac{\%\text{ dose as debrisoquine}}{\%\text{ dose as 4-hydroxydebrisoquine}}$$

Poor hydroxylators have ratio > 20.
Extensive hydroxylators have ratio < 12.5.

Inheritance. Poor hydroxylation is autosomal recessive.

Prevalence. Poor hydroxylators: U.K.   9%
                                       Arabs   1%
                                       Hong Kong Chinese   30%

Drugs with metabolism associated with debrisoquine 4-hydroxylation
Metoprolol; Timolol; Propranolol
Phenformin
Phenytoin
Perhexiline
Encainide

Clinical relevance
1. Oxidation status determines efficacy.
2. Phenformin lactic acidosis occurs in poor metabolisers.
3. Vertigo and confusion after nortriptyline commoner in poor metabolisers.
4. Possibly captopril-induced agranulocytosis commoner in poor metabolisers.

b. *N-oxidation of sparteine* (uterine stimulant used in Germany). Based on 0–12 h urine sample after 100 mg sparteine sulphate.

$$\text{Metabolic ratio} = \frac{\%\text{ dose excreted as sparteine}}{\%\text{ dose as sparteine metabolites}}$$

Non-inheritors have log (metabolic ratio) ≈ 32.
Inheritance. Non-metabolism is autosomal recessive.
Prevalence. Non-metabolism: Canadian Chinese 30%
                               Canadians of European origin 5%

Relationship to debrisoquine polymorphism. Both determined by relative amount of form of hepatic cytochrome P450. May be closely related but not identical cytochromes since in a few people there is discordance between debrisoquine and sparteine phenotypes.

Suxamethonium sensitivity

Suxamethonium-induced muscular paralysis usually lasts 5–10 mins due to rapid hydrolysis of drug by plasma pseudocholinesterase. Several variants of enzyme described, some of which cause prolonged paralysis requiring mechanical ventilation for some hours. Most common variant is $E_1^a E_1^a$ inherited as autosomal recessive (1 in 2500 in UK but absent in Japanese and Eskimos, rare in Africans).

Variants in suxamethonium sensitivity

Genotype	Phenotype	Prevalence	Response to suxamethonium
$E_1^u E_1^u$	Usual type of esterase	96%	Normal
$E_1^a E_1^u$	Some decreased sensitivity to inhibitors dibucaine and fluoride	1/26	Normal
$E_1^a E_1^a$	Greatly decreased sensitivity to dibucaine and fluoride	1/2800	Prolonged
$E_1^f E_1^u$	Some decreased sensitivity to fluoride	1/280	Normal
$E_1^f E_1^f$	Greatly decreased sensitivity to fluoride	1/300 000	Prolonged
$E_1^s E_1^u$	Some reduction in enzymic activity	1/190	Normal or almost normal
$E_1^s E_1^s$	No enzymic activity	1/140 000 (1% of Eskimos)	Grossly prolonged
$E_1^a E_1^f$	Decreased sensitivity to dibucaine and fluoride	1/29 000	Prolonged
$E_1^a E_1^s$	Greatly decreased sensitivity to dibucaine and fluoride	1/20 000	Grossly prolonged
$E_1^f E_1^s$	Decreased sensitivity to dibucaine and fluoride	1/200 000	Prolonged
$E_1^+ E_1^+$	30% increase in enzyme activity	1/10	Shortened
$E_{Cynthiana}$	2–3 × increase in enzyme activity	Unknown	Resistance to drug

Drug excretion

Dubin–Johnson's syndrome: failure of excretion of bilirubin glucuronide into bile; inherited as autosomal recessive. Jaundice can be precipitated or worsened by oral contraceptives.

DISCONTINUOUS VARIATION IN DRUG RESPONSE

Glucose 6-phosphate dehydrogenase (G6PD) deficiency

Inheritance

Sex-linked (X chromosome) defect of intermediate dominance
determining activity of G6PD. Affects about 100 million people in
world: African Negroes; some Mediterranean races; Kurdish and Iraqi
Jews; some Filipinos; Chinese and S.E. Asians.

Heterozygous females have 2 red cell populations (+ and −
enzyme), proportion varies from 1–99% sensitive-cells: approximately
$\frac{1}{3}$ heterozygous females have sufficiently high fraction of affected cells
to show haemolysis.

Mutation has survived in its areas of distribution because it confers
resistance to malaria.

Mechanism

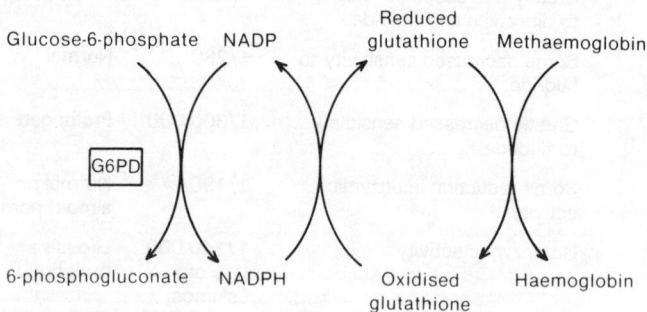

Fig. 3.1

G6PD activity maintains low levels of methaemoglobin in red cells.
If methaemoglobin level increases, haemolysis occurs.

Clinical features

Over 100 variants G6PD described. Two common types in the UK:

a. African type A — normal amount of enzyme but rapid decline
   in activity as red cells age
   — suffer mild enzyme deficiency with 8–20%
   normal activity. Have haemolysis on drug
   challenge.

b. Mediterranean type — severe (0–4% normal) enzyme activity
   deficit
   — mild chronic haemolytic anaemia with
   severe haemolysis after drug challenge.

RBC reduced glutathione (GSH) diminished in deficiency of:
　glucose 6-phosphate dehydrogenase (G6PD)
　γ-glutamylcysteine synthetase
　glutathione reductase
　glutathione peroxidase.

and may result in haemolysis when the following are administered:
　analgesics — aspirin
　antimalarials — primaquine, pamaquine, quinine, chloroquine
　antibacterials — sulphonamides, sulphones, nitrofurantoin,
　　　　　　　　 chloramphenicol, PAS
　miscellaneous — quinidine, vitamin K, Fava bean.

Porphyrias

Metabolic disorders characterised by tissue accumulation of porphyrins and/or precursors with characteristics symptoms. Some types have specific enzyme deficiencies; others as yet of uncertain mechanism. In general, increased levels of δ-aminolaevulinic acid (ALA) and porphobilinogen (PBG) associated with acute attacks and porphyrins with photosensitivity.

Acute attacks bear a superficial resemblance to lead poisoning and comprise:
　Abdominal symptoms — colic, constipation, nausea, vomiting.
　Psychiatric abnormalities — restlessness, confusion, psychosis.
　Neurological features — peripheral neuropathy, paralysis or paresis of limbs, respiratory paralysis (commonest cause of death), rarely seizures.
　Lesions occur at several points of porphyrin metabolism.

Acute attacks occur intermittently and ascribed to increased ALA synthetase activity which exacerbates biochemical abnormalities. Drugs (and endogenous steroids) commonest precipitating factors.
　Acute attacks occur in:

1. Acute intermittent porphyria (Swedish type — commonest in UK). Autosomal dominant inheritance of uroporphyrinogen synthetase deficiency. Rare before puberty and commoner in women often presenting in pregnancy due to increased steroid.
2. Hereditary coproporphyria. Rare. Autosomal dominant inheritance of partial deficiency of coproporphyrin oxygenase.
3. Variegate porphyria (South African type — 3/1000 but occurs in Europe — George III probably had it). Autosomal dominant but deficit obscure — ferrochelatase may be unstable or deficient or possibly there is block of coproporphyrin metabolism.

Drugs which can precipitate acute porphyria attacks
Hypnosedatives: barbiturates (including anaesthetic
　　　　　　　 barbiturates), chlordiazepoxide
Anticonvulsants: phenytoin, succinimides
Oral hypoglycaemics: chlorpropamide, tolbutamide

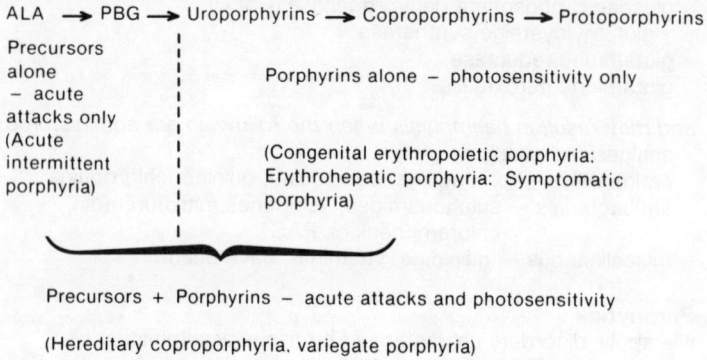

ALA ⟶ PBG ⟶ Uroporphyrins ⟶ Coproporphyrins ⟶ Protoporphyrins

Precursors
alone
– acute   Porphyrins alone – photosensitivity only
attacks only
(Acute
intermittent   (Congenital erythropoietic porphyria:
porphyria)   Erythrohepatic porphyria: Symptomatic
                             porphyria)

Precursors + Porphyrins – acute attacks and photosensitivity

(Hereditary coproporphyria. variegate porphyria)

Fig. 3.2

Antimicrobials: chloramphenicol, chloroquine, griseofulvin
Steroids: oestrogens, oral contraceptive pill.

Steroid-induced raised intraocular pressure
Chronic use of steroid eye drops produces raised intraocular pressure
in genetically predisposed.

	0–5	5–15	15+
Increase in intraocular pressure on exposure to 1% dexamethasone eye drops (mmHg)			
Percentage of white population	66	29	5
Proposed genotype — autosomal recessive inheritance	P^LP^L	P^LP^H	P^HP^H
Chance of ultimate development of open angle glaucoma in later life (compared with P^LP^L individuals)	1	18	101

Table 1 Discontinuous variation in drug response

Pharmacogenetic variation	Mechanism	Inheritance	Occurrence	Drugs involved	Effects
Haemoglobin H (a form of α-thalassaemia)	HbH is a β chain tetramer, which tends to form Met Hb with oxidising drugs	Autosomal recessive	1/300 in Thailand	As is G6PD deficiency	Drug-induced haemolytic anaemia. Heinz bodies
HbM	Met HbM is resistant to Met Hb reductase	Autosomal dominant		Nitrites, nitrates, chlorates, phenacetin,	Met Hb cyanosis on drug exposure
Hereditary methaemoglobinaemia	Reductase deficiency	Autosomal recessive (but heterozygotes show some response)	1/100 are heterozygotes	acetanilide, sulphonamides, dapsone, primaquine	Met Hb cyanosis on drug exposure
Hb Zurich Hb Köln Hb Hammersmith	Unstable Hb which readily forms Heinz bodies		Rare	Sulphonamides, primaquine	Drug-induced haemolysis
Warfarin resistance	Reduced affinity of vitamin K expoxide reductase for warfarin	Autosomal dominant	Rare	Warfarin, dicoumarol, phenindione	5–20 times the usual dose of drug required to anticoagulate

Table 1 (continued)

Pharmacogenetic variation	Mechanism	Inheritance	Occurrence	Drugs involved	Effects
Chloramphenicol-induced bone marrow depression	Idiosyncratic inhibition of DNA synthesis in marrow cells	Probably genetically determined	Rare	Chloramphenicol	Severe, often irreversible, aplasia of bone marrow
Increased sensitivity to ethanol	Unknown central factors. Increased peripheral autonomic sensitivity	Racial	Common in Oriental races	Ethanol	Increased flushing, increased intoxication
Intravascular clotting with oral contraceptives	Unknown	Strong association with blood groups A and AB	Rare	Oestrogen-containing preparations	Increased risk of venous and arterial thrombosis
Atropine sensitivity	Low vagal tone or increased sensitivity to sympathetic effects	Trisomy 21 and other forms of Down's syndrome	Common in Down's syndrome	Atropine and other anticholinergics	Tachycardia and other signs atropine toxicity
Malignant hyperthermia	Defect in Ca^{++} storing with muscle fibre	Autosomal dominant	1/20 000	Nitrous oxide, halothane, ether, cyclopropane, suxamethonium	Hyperthermia, rigidity, metabolic acidosis, Treat with dantrolene

Table 2 Discontinuous variation in drug metabolism

Pharmacogenetic variation	Mechanism	Inheritance	Occurrence	Drugs involved	Effects
Acatalasia	Lack of r.b.c. catalase	Autosomal recessive	Up to 1% in some Japanese populations	Hydrogen peroxide	Approx 50% suffer recurrent sepsis of mouth and pharynx
Slow metabolism of tolbutamide	Impaired metabolic inactivation (possibly same as defective carbon oxidation of debrisoquine)	Autosomal recessive	? same as defective metabolism of debrisoquine	Tolbutamide	Increased drug effect with usual doses
Unresponsiveness to purine antimetabolites	Lack of hypoxanthine guanine phosphoribosyl transferase (HGPRT), therefore fails to activate drugs to nucleotide analogues	1. Lesch–Nyhan syndrome: X-linked recessive 2. Some forms of gout: X-linked recessive		6-mercaptopurine 6-thioguanine 8-azaguanine azathioprine	Lack of anticancer activity
Ethanol: 1. Rapid metabolisers	Variant hyperactive form of ADH 2	Autosomal	4–20% Europeans	Ethanol	40–50% more rapid metabolism

Table 2 (continued)

Pharmacogenetic variation	Mechanism	Inheritance	Occurrence	Drugs involved	Effects
2. Racial differences	Unknown	?	?	Ethanol	Rate of alcohol metabolism: Europeans 0.145 g/kg/h; Eskimos 0.110 g/kg/h; Red Indians 0.101 g/kg/h
Impairment of bilirubin conjugation:	Lack of UDP glucuronyl transferase. Failure of drug conjugation and thus impairment of excretion.			Paracetamol Tetrahydrocortisol Menthol Chloral hydrate Trichloroethanol Salicylamide	Impaired drug glucuronidation
1. Crigler-Najjar syndrome	Complete enzyme lack	Autosomal recessive			
2. Moderate impairment of conjugation	Inducible enzyme present	Autosomal dominant with incomplete penetration			
3. Gilbert's syndrome	Inducible enzyme present	Autosomal dominant			

4. Drugs at the extremes of age

DRUGS AND INFANTS AND CHILDREN

1/6 newborns in special care nurseries ⎤
3/5 children in hospital ⎦ receive drug therapy

Incidence of adverse effects (10–15%) similar to adults in children but higher (25%) in neonates.

Children not miniature adults in terms of drug handling because of differences in body constitution. For example:

1. Body water (as % body weight)

	Neonate	Adult
Total	75	60

2. Renal function — changes in clearance (ml/min)

	Infant	Adult
GFR	10	130

Adult GFR attained 3–5 months.

3. Hepatic enzyme activity low in neonates for some systems, e.g. chloramphenicol glucuronyl transferase, but not others, e.g. sulphation of paracetamol.

4. GI function very different in terms of transit time, enzymes etc. in neonates, e.g.

	Neonate	Adult
Gastric emptying time (mins)	87	65
Gastric acid output (mmol/10 kg/hr)	0.15	2

5. Ratio of surface area/body weight

	Weight (kg)	Surface area (m^2)	Ratio (kg/m^2)
Neonate	1.5	0.13	11.5
Adult	70	1.8	39

Dosing related to surface area most physiological dose adjustment rule, but doses usually calculated accordingly to body weight.

However if body surface area (BSA) is to be used then approximate dose for patient is

$$\frac{BSA(m^2)}{1.8} \times \text{adult dose}$$

Pharmacokinetic effects

1. *Absorption*: Reduced gastric acidity in neonates results in greater oral absorption of ampicillin, flucloxacillin, amoxycillin as compared to adults. Neonates absorb phenobarbitone and vitamin E poorly but digoxin, diazepam and cotrimoxazole normally absorbed.

Generally neonatal GI drug absorption is clinically adequate.

Older infants and children absorb some drugs, e.g. diazepam, clonazepam, sodium valproate more rapidly but with same bioavailability as adults.

Absorption from i.m. injections in neonates may be erratic for some drugs, e.g. gentamicin, digoxin.

Infant skin is thin and percutaneous absorption is good, e.g. steroid creams (→ Cushing's); topical sulphonamide mafenide (→ methaemoglobinaemia); hexachlorophane (→ neurotoxicity).

2. *Distribution*: Fat content is low in children.

	Fat as % body weight
Premature	3
Neonate (full term)	12
Age 1 year	30
Age 18 years	18

V_d of fat soluble drugs, e.g. diazepam thus lower in babies than adults.

Plasma protein binding of drugs reduced in neonates due to 20% (approx) lower albumin conc and altered capacity so V_d rises.

Blood-brain barrier more permeable in neonates than older children and adults, e.g. opiates, penicillin.

3. *Metabolism*: Liver volume/kg decreases after birth into adult years. Some (but not all) enzyme systems less active in neonates but many increase (relatively) in children.

Previous intrauterine or postnatal drug exposure can affect neonatal metabolism, e.g. phenobarbitone reduces neonatal diazepam $T_{1/2}$ to 12–15 hours.

Chloramphenicol produces 'grey baby' syndrome in neonates due to high plasma levels as elimination delayed by inefficient glucuronidization.

4. *Excretion*: All renal mechanisms (filtration, secretion, reabsorption) are reduced in babies — filtration is also relatively more important than other mechanisms as compared with adults.

In general, renal excretion of drugs is less in neonates compared to older patients. GFR rapidly increases after a few weeks and doses of drugs excreted this way, e.g. aminoglycosides, penicillins should be increased after first week of life.

Drug prescribing in infancy
1. Minimum number of drugs for shortest time (as always!).
2. If possible use drugs with high therapeutic index, available kinetic information in children and possibility of drug level monitoring if required.
3. Liquid oral preparations for young children (if available) but can often swallow tablets or capsules. Chronic use of sucrose-containing elixirs may cause caries and gingivitis.
4. Drugs should not be added to milk in infant feeding bottles since interaction could occur or dosage may be reduced if feed not taken completely.
5. In general, rectal administration is erratic and may upset older children so is discouraged but can be useful if child is vomiting or convulsing.
6. Dosage is critical especially in first 30 days (neonate). Ideally, use surface area (see above) except for prematures when it is inaccurate. For drugs with a high therapeutic index age can be used according to:

Age	% adult dose
Premature	Not applicable
1 month	12.5
2 months	15
4 months	20
1 year	25
3 years	33
7 years	50
12 years	75

Dosing by weight often useful but in obesity need to dose in terms of ideal body weight (from age and height).

DRUGS DURING PREGNANCY

Average number of drugs taken during pregnancy — 4.2 (Scotland 1972): not including those taken during labour.

Embryo more susceptible to adverse drug effects than at any other period of life. All drugs can cross placenta if given in sufficient quantity. Effects may be:
1. fetal death and abortion

2. malformations
3. affect postnatal behaviour, e.g. sedation; withdrawal syndrome
4. produce malignancy in later life.

Major risk of malformation is up to 8th week postconception (i.e. often before pregnancy diagnosed) but adverse effects occur after this.

Drug	Possible effect on fetus	Trimester
Androgens	Masculinisation of female	1, 2, 3
Stilboestrol	Vaginal adenocarcinoma in adult life	1
Methotrexate	Malformation and abortion	1
Anticonvulsants	Cleft hip and other malformations	1
Salicylates	Risk of haemorrhage in neonate, intrauterine closure of ductus, delayed onset of labour	3
Retinoids	Congenital malformations	1, 2, 3
Benzodiazepines	Neonatal drowsiness, hypotonia, withdrawal syndrome	3
Warfarin	Choanal atresia, fetal and neonatal haemorrhage	1, 2, 3
Alcohol	Fetal alcohol syndrome, growth retardation, withdrawal syndrome	1, 2, 3
Aminoglycosides	Auditory and vestibular nerve damage	2, 3

NB Thalidomide (no longer available) produced malformations in about 25% pregnancies.

Rule Drugs should *only* be used during pregnancy if of proven benefit to mother of fetus and with due consideration of risks. *Any* woman of child-bearing age may become pregnant!

DRUGS IN BREAST MILK

Many drugs enter breast milk — usually small amounts and not harmful.

Entry depends upon pH and pK_a of drug — lipid soluble drugs diffuse in as their non-ionised form. Milk has lower pH than plasma so concentrates weak bases; weak acids usually at lower concentration than plasma.

Only occasionally do drugs in milk adversely affect infant, examples:

Drug given to mother	Effect on baby
Benzodiazepines	Lethargy, weight loss
Chlorpromazine	Drowsiness
Lithium	Hypotonia, hypothermia, cyanosis
Senna, danthron	Diarrhoea
Chloramphenicol	Bone marrow depression
Ephedrine	Irritability and sleep disturbances
Aspirin	Reye's syndrome

DRUGS AND THE ELDERLY

10% of geriatric admissions are associated with drug-related problems, because:
1. Elderly receive more drugs than young. Several illnesses may coexist. 2/3 receive 1–3 drugs and 1/3 4–6 + drugs simultaneously.
2. Non-compliance in elderly is 50–60% of which half is serious (omitting necessary drugs or taking inappropriate drugs). 20% due to lack of knowledge of drug regimen; 20% due to taking drugs not currently prescribed.
3. Increased sensitivity of aged to drugs and adverse effects.
4. Incorrect and harmful use of drugs, e.g. prochlorperazine for loss of postural stability.

Increased sensitivity to drugs
A. Pharmacokinetic effects
1. Absorption. Little evidence of major alteration in absorption.
2. Distribution. Aging accompanied by relative increase in fat, reduced water, muscles mass and body weight.
   Plasma protein changes may occur with decreased albumin and increased gamma globulin but no defect in drug binding affinity found.

Increased V_d	Decreased V_d
Benzodiazepines	Digoxin
Chlormethiazole	Ethanol
Gentamicin	

3. Metabolism. Elderly have:
a. Altered hepatic metabolism but only in some cases, eg:

Reduced clearance	Unchanged clearance
Diazepam — oxidation	Temazepam — glucuronidation
Propranolol — oxidation	Warfarin — oxidation
Nortriptyline — oxidation	Lignocaine — oxidation

b. Decreased hepatic blood flow. Suggests main effect of aging is on Phase I metabolism — 40–50% reduction (mainly due to reduced cardiac output): could affect highly cleared drugs like propranolol.
c. Reduced capacity for microsomal enzyme induction following inducing agents. Also elderly smoke and drink less than young so hepatic enzymes less induced.

No effects found on non-microsomally metabolised drugs like alcohol, isoniazid, aspirin.
4. *Excretion*. The most important factor is that glomerular filtration rate falls with age. GFR ≃ 153 – 0.96 (Age).

Tubular secretion also declines.

Deficits greatly worsen during acute illness

B. *Pharmacodynamic effects*

Much of the increased sensitivity of elderly explained by altered pharmacokinetics but may also show altered response although as yet little information available. Examples:
1. Elderly show greater CNS depression and confusion with sedating drugs.
2. Warfarin produces greater inhibition of hepatic clotting factor synthesis in the old than in the young.
3. Increased sensitivity to β-blockers with age may reflect reduced β-adrenoceptor density. Reduced doses of digoxin are required.
4. Increased frequency and magnitude of drug-induced postural hypotension probably results from age-related impairment of baroreceptor reflexes.
5. Antimuscarinics more likely to cause constipation, urinary retention, hallucinations and aggravation of glaucoma.

Drug usage in the aged
Many of these rules apply at all ages.
1. Use the fewest drugs and the simplest regime possible.
2. Use the lowest dose.
3. Do not use drugs to treat symptoms without knowing their cause.
4. Discontinue a drug if it becomes unnecessary.
5. Do not withhold drugs because of old age but remember drugs cannot cure old age.

5. Effect of disease on pharmacokinetics

RENAL IMPAIRMENT

Reduction in the dose of drugs is needed in patients with renal failure if elimination of the drug is mainly renal or if toxicity is poorly tolerated or if the drug is toxic at elevated blood levels.

In renal failure, drugs eliminated by the kidney will have an extended half-life, thus steady state blood levels will be delayed ($T_{1/2} \times 5$) and a loading dose will be needed.

Particular care should be taken to avoid potentially nephrotoxic drugs.

Overall drug elimination rate (k) is sum of the rates for renal (kr) and non-renal (nr) elimination.

$$k = kr + knr$$

For most drugs kr is also proportional to creatinine clearance (CL_{cr})

$$kr \propto CL_{cr}$$

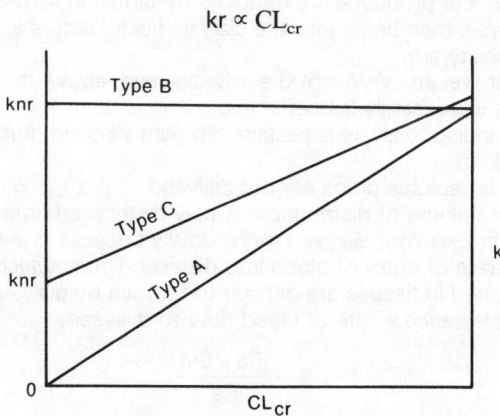

Fig. 5.1

so k = α CL$_{cr}$ where α is a proportionality constant and k = α CL$_{cr}$ + knr.

If k is plotted against CL$_{cr}$ (the Dettli nomogram) the ordinate intercept will be knr and three classes of drugs can be distinguished.
Type A: drugs entirely dependent upon renal function for elimination, e.g. gentamicin, kanamycin and other aminoglycosides; cephaloridine, cephalexin, lithium.
Type B: drugs entirely dependent upon non-renal routes (e.g. hepatic) for elimination, e.g. adriamycin, corticosteroids, chloramphenicol, diazepam, propranolol, rifampicin.
Type C: drugs dependent upon both renal and non-renal routes of elimination, e.g. digoxin, ethambutol, methyldopa, methotrexate, procainamide.

Type B drugs require no change in regime unless renally excreted active metabolites are involved. Type A and C drugs require dosage modification. This can be done using a Dettli nomogram since k for normal renal function and knr are known for many drugs.

Pharmacodynamic changes
Remember some drug effects, without importance in normal renal function, may become significant in renal failure, e.g.:
1. tetracycline, glucocorticoids (raise urea due to anti-anabolic effects)
2. carbenoxolone, and NSAID (salt and water retention)
3. benzodiazepines, barbiturates, phenothiazines and opioids (produce CNS depression in renal failure)
4. digoxin, nitrofurantoin (nausea).

Dialysis
Drugs (like waste products) are removed by diffusion across the artificial dialysis membrane into the dialysis fluid. Factors affecting drug dialysability are:
1. Molecular weight: MW < 500 easily dialysed, above this it becomes increasingly less effective.
2. Protein binding: dialysis is passive, so tightly bound drugs not removed.
3. Polarity: fat-soluble drugs are not dialysed.
4. Apparent volume of distribution: widely distributed drugs, e.g. digoxin, imipramine, dialysed more slowly because rate-limiting factor is rate of entry of blood into dialyser. Drugs which are concentrated in tissues are difficult to remove by dialysis.
   Dialysis clearance $\propto$ rate of blood flow to dialyser

$$= \frac{(Ca - Cv)}{Ca}$$

Ca = arterial drug concentration (entering dialyser)
Cv = venous drug concentration (leaving dialyser)
(Note similarity to expression for hepatic clearance)

CARDIAC FAILURE

Absorption
1. Reduced gut mobility (increased sympathetic activity)
2. Mucosal oedema
3. Reduced blood flow to gut.
   May result in reduced GI absorption of some drugs, e.g. hydrochlorothiazide, frusemide, procainamide.

Distribution
Reduced tissue blood flow changes distribution;
   Apparent volume of distribution reduced for quinidine, lignocaine, procainamide. May result in higher toxicity. Frusemide becomes less effective because lower urine concentration.

Metabolism
1. Blood flow to liver falls in proportion to cardiac output.
2. Hepatic metabolic capacity reduced by hepatocellular damage due to hypoperfusion or congestion and hypoxaemia.
   May result in higher levels with increased toxicity of drugs with high extraction ratio, e.g. lignocaine

Excretion
Renal clearance affected by:
1. Decreased glomerular filtration rate resulting from hypoperfusion.
2. Increased reabsorption due to altered intrarenal blood flow.
   Examples: procainamide, digoxin.

HEPATIC DISEASE

Difficulties due to:
1. Impaired drug metabolism or reduced excretion into bile (e.g. rifampicin, fusidic acid).
2. Hypoalbuminaemia increases the effects of highly protein bound drugs (e.g. phenytoin).
3. Reduced synthesis of clotting factors increases sensitivity to oral anticoagulants (e.g. warfarin).
4. Hepatic encephalopathy and other cerebral disturbances are readily provoked by sedatives, opioids, potassium losing diuretics, constipating drugs.
5. Oedema made worse by NSAID and corticosteroids.
   Liver plays central role in drug elimination but liver disease produces effects on drug disposition which are often difficult to interpret. This is because of different functional effects, e.g.

Disease	Hepatic blood flow	Hepatocellular mass	Hepatocyte function
Cirrhosis			
— moderate	↓	Unchanged	Unchanged
— severe	↓ ↓	↓	
Viral hepatitis	Unchanged or ↑	Unchanged or ↓	↓
Alcoholic hepatitis	Unchanged or ↓	Variable	↓

Changes in intrinsic free drug clearance (CL_{int})
Examples of reduced intrinsic clearance:
Cirrhosis: theophylline, diazepam
Hepatitis: diazepam. But no effect on warfarin, phenytoin, tolbutamide.
Some routes, e.g. glucuronidation, apparently less sensitive to pathological changes than others.

Changes in hepatic blood flow
Clearance of highly extracted drugs depends upon hepatic blood flow. Alteration in flow patterns may occur with *intra- and extra-hepatic shunting* of blood away from metabolising liver cells (so-called 'intact hepatocyte' theory) and 60% or more of portal blood can be diverted from functioning hepatotcytes. This can alter hepatic first-pass metabolism after oral drug administration. These effects contribute to increased bioavailability in cirrhosis of chlormethiazole (10 × increase); pethidine, pentazocine, labetalol, propranolol.

Clinical implications
Conventional liver function tests have poor predictive function in relation to drug metabolism. Best warning indicators are low serum albumin (< 30 g/l) and/or increased prothrombin time. Fortunately the liver has remarkable functional reserves and damage is usually severe before important changes occur and even then these are usually no greater than 2 or 3-fold. Some individuals may show greater effects but the inter-patient variability in drug effects is often greater than this in the absence of liver disease.
    Few generalisations can be made about drug handling in liver disease:
1. Often no need to modify drug regimes specifically because of liver disease: more important to be aware of dangers and to react appropriately using plasma level monitoring and/or clinical skills.
2. Avoid known hepatoxic drugs.
3. Use drugs eliminated via non-hepatic routes.
4. Avoid drugs requiring hepatic activation, e.g. prednisone.

GASTROINTESTINAL DISEASE

Rarely major effect on absorption, e.g. protein losing enteropathy. Some examples of other mechanisms:

Gastrointestinal factor	Drug whose absorption is altered
1. Achlorhydria (also alters rate of stomach emptying)	↓ — aspirin, cephalexin ↑ — benzylpenicillin
2. Gastrectomy	↓ — levodopa, quinidine, ethambutol, sulphonamides, iron ↑ — digoxin
3. Coeliac disease	↓ — amoxycillin, pivampicillin, thyroxin ↑ — cephalexin, clindamycin, sulphamethoxazole, trimethoprim, propranolol
4. Crohn's disease	↑ — sulphamethoxazole — propranolol Delayed peak trimethoprim and lincomycin
5. Pancreatic disease	↓ — Vitamins A, D, K; cephalexin; phenoxymethylpenicillin

Note: Malabsorption syndromes, coeliac disease etc. have variable and unpredictable effects on drug absorption. Treatment may alter response, e.g. phenoxymethylpenicillin absorption decreased in untreated coeliac disease but normal after 8 months gluten-free diet.

6. Adverse drug reactions and interactions

Adverse drug reactions: unintended effects of substances used in prevention, diagnosis or treatment of disease.
Occur in — 10–15% hospital in-patients
— 40% patients in general practice
Responsible for 3–5% hospital admissions.
1 in 1000 medical in-patients in USA may die as consequence but only 1 in 10 is preventable.
Rational use of the *minimum number of drugs* per patient is simplest way to avoid adverse drug effects.

Thompson/Rawlins Classification

	Type A	Type B
Pharmacology	Augmented	Bizarre
Predictable	Yes	No
Dose-dependent	Yes	No
Morbidity	High	Low
Mortality	Low	High

Examples:

Phenytoin	Sedation, cerebellar signs; enzyme induction.	Rashes; Pseudolymphoma.
Amitriptyline	Anticholinergic effects; sedation; sensitivity to pressor amines.	Hepatotoxicity.

Type A reactions — in individuals lying at extremes of dose-response curve, occur for 3 reasons:
1. Pharmaceutical — differences in bioavailability of preparations produce effects in the predisposed.
2. Pharmacokinetic — individual differences in absorption, distribution, metabolism, excretion result in toxicity.
3. Pharmacodynamic — individual differences in target organ susceptibility.

Type B reactions — qualitatively abnormal effects apparently unrelated to drug's known actions occur for 3 reasons:

1. Pharmaceutical — idiosyncratic response to non-drug components of drug products, e.g. tartrazine (yellow food dye: asthma), lactose (GI intolerance) or storage degradation products, e.g. of tetracycline (renal tubular damage).
2. Pharmacokinetic — theoretical possibility of formation of novel metabolites or of antigenic complexes.
3. Pharmacodynamic — altered target organ responses, e.g. G6PD deficiency, porphyria, allergic responses to drugs which are not intrinsically antigenic.

Drug interactions
Pharmacological responses which cannot be explained by the action of a single drug but are due to two or more drugs acting simultaneously.
May be harmful by:
1. increasing toxicity
2. decreasing efficacy.
OR
beneficial by allowing reduction of dose by enhanced efficacy without increased toxicity.
OR
harmless.

Incidence
— Increased by number of drugs taken, e.g. with 2–5 drugs 19% incidence of potential interactions; with 6 + drugs incidence is 80 + %.
— Occur in 0.5–2% hospital in-patients.
— Significance of such figures in clinical practice difficult to determine: not every patient at risk is affected; many isolated case reports exist without validation.

Mechanisms of interactions
1. *Pharmaceutical incompatibility outside the body.*
2. *Pharmacokinetic*
a. *Drug absorption — examples:*

Mixture	Mechanism	Effect
Tetracycline + Ca^{++}, Fe^{++}, Al^{+++}, Mg^{++}	Chelation	Mutually reduced absorption
Anticoagulants } thyroxine } + Cholestyramine	Binding to resin	Reduced drug absorption

b. *Drug distribution* — displacement from protein binding often suggested as cause of interaction but rarely proven. In some cases, e.g. phenylbutazone + warfarin interaction, inhibition of warfarin metabolism seems more likely. Suggested displacement interactions include:

Bound drug	Displacing drug	Result
Bilirubin	Sulphonamides	Kernicterus
	Vitamin K	
Tolbutamide	Salicylates	Hypoglycaemia
	Phenylbutazone	
Warfarin	Salicylates	Haemorrhage
	Trichloroacetic acid	
	Clofibrate	

Altered drug uptake at site of action:

Primary drug	Inhibition drug	Effect of interaction
Guanethidine	Tricyclic	Reduction of
Bethanidine	antidepressants;	hypotensive effect
Debrisoquine	Phenothiazines,	
Clonidine		
Phenylephrine	Tricyclic	Potentiation of
Adrenaline	antidepressants;	pressor effect of
Noradrenaline		catecholamines

c. *Drug metabolism* — enzyme induction by increasing drug inactivation may produce tolerance or completely nullify drug action. Examples include:

Primary drug	Inducing agent	Effect of interaction
Oral anticoagulants	Barbiturates	Decreased
e.g. warfarin	Dichloralphenazone	anticoagulation
	Rifampicin	
Tolbutamide	Phenytoin	Decreased
		hypoglycaemia
Oral contraceptives	Carbamazepine	Pregnancy
Prednisolone	Carbamazepine	Reduced steroid levels

Alternatively some drugs may act as enzyme inhibitors and raise the concentration of concurrently administered drugs. Examples:

Primary drug	Inhibiting drug	Effect of interaction
Phenytoin	Isoniazid	Phenytoin intoxication
Oral anticoagulants	Allopurinol	Haemorrhage
Tolbutamide	Phenylbutazone	Hypoglycaemia
Chlorpropamide	Chloramphenicol	
6-mercaptopurine	Allopurinol	Bone marrow
Azathioprine		suppression

d. *Drug excretion*: may be changed by drugs which alter urinary pH. Alternatively drugs may compete for active renal tubular secretion — examples:

Primary drug	Competing drug	Effect of interaction
Penicillin	Probenecid	Increased penicillin blood level
Methotrexate	Salicylates	Bone marrow suppression
Salicylate	Probenecid	Salicylate toxicity
Indomethacin	Probenecid	Indomethacin toxicity
Lithium	Thiazide diuretics	Lithium toxicity
Digoxin	Spironolactone	Increased plasma digoxin levels

3. *Pharmacodynamic interactions* at drug receptor sites or by secondary physiological mechanisms. These may be **synergistic**:

Primary drug	Interacts with	Resulting in
Alcohol	Other CNS depressant drugs e.g. hyoscine antihistamines opioids	CNS depression
Tubocurarine	Aminoglycosides Quinidine	Prolonged paralysis
Oral hypoglycaemic drugs	Salicylates Propranolol	Prolonged or excessive hypoglycaemia
Digitalis	Propranolol	Bradycardia due to unopposed vagal effects of glycoside
Antihypertensive drugs	Diuretics	Enhanced hypotension
Ergotamine	Propranolol	Excessive vasoconstriction

Or **antagonistic**:

Primary drug	Interacts with	Resulting in
β-adrenoceptor agonists	β-adrenoceptor antagonists	Antagonism of bronchodilator effects
Methotrexate	Folinic acid	Antagonism of toxic (and possibly antineoplastic) effects of methotrexate
Opiates	Naloxone	Reversal of opiate effects

Primary drug	Interacts with	Resulting in
Warfarin	Oestrogens	Warfarin effect antagonised by increased clotting factor synthesis
Hypotensive drugs	Non-steroidal anti-inflammatory agents	Antagonism of hypotensive effect due to sodium retention

Important drug–drug interactions
Occur with drugs that have steep dose-response curve, i.e. small changes in dose produce large pharmacological effects:
  anticoagulants
  oral hypoglycaemic drugs
  anticonvulsants
  antiarrhythmics
  cardiac glycosides
  antihypertensives
  drugs acting on the CNS, e.g. alcohol, MAOI.

7. Drug development and adverse reaction monitoring

DRUG DEVELOPMENT

Takes up to 10 years.
Costs approximately $100 million to develop new drug to marketing stage.

Pre-clinical development
Research policy decision
↓
Synthesis of new chemical entities (NCE) based on:
1. random synthesis of new compounds
2. structural variation of compounds with known pharmacological activity.
↓
Animal pharmacology to:
1. define pharmacology
2. define toxicity
   a. short term studies in at least two species, one not being a rodent
   b. reproductive and teratology studies
   c. mutagenicity and carcinogenicity studies.

Clinical development
About 1 in 1000 NCE reach this stage
If decided to proceed with development, studies along several lines:
1. Pharmaceutical — stability
               — formulation
               — compatibility with other tablet/infusion ingredients
2. Pharmacological — further chronic animal toxicity
                 — initial animal metabolic and pharmacokinetic studies
                 — development of assay
3. Clinical pharmacology studies divided into four phases:

Phase I — first time into man to determine actions and toxic effects. Pharmacokinetics usually studied at this stage.

(i) Ethical Committee permission required but if in volunteers CSM is not involved.
(ii) Usually fully-informed normal volunteers but if drug likely to be toxic, e.g. anti-cancer agent, then patients with poor prognosis may volunteer.
(iii) Dose ranging single rising dose study beginning with 1/50 to 1/100 the effective dose in animals and increasing until desired effect or toxicity found. Extensive biochemical, haematological and physiological tests conducted.
(iv) If (iii) satisfactory followed by chronic (7–14 day) administration
In experienced hands is relatively safe: one clinically significant medical event every 9600 days of subject exposure in one 10-year study of Phase I experiments.

Phase II — is drug therapeutically useful?
Requires Clinical Trial Certificate (CTC) or Exemption (CTE) from CSM as well as Ethical Committee permission.
(i) Initially open, uncontrolled, dose-ranging studies in volunteer patients. Later controlled studies under single-or double-blind conditions with comparisons with inert placebo or standard drugs are included.
(ii) Involve perhaps 100–500 patients only.

Phase III — larger trials to compare new drug with existing ones.
To establish profile of efficacy and toxicity.
Requires CTC/CTE and Ethical Committee permission.
(i) Many centres and/or multi-centre.
(ii) Double-blind, placebo or active drug controlled trials commonly used. Patients must be informed of participation in trial and given full details.
(iii) Involves 250–2000 patients only.

Phase IV — subsequent observations — including postmarketing surveillance.

Drug regulation in UK
Ministers of Health and Agriculture (for veterinary products) responsible for administration of Medicines Act (1968) are advised by (amongst others):
1. Committee on Safety of Medicines (CSM)
2. Committee on Review of Medicines — to review all marketed medicines.
3. British Pharmacopoeia Committee — draw up new editions. The drug regulatory body is part of the Department of Health and has the structure shown in Figure 7.1.

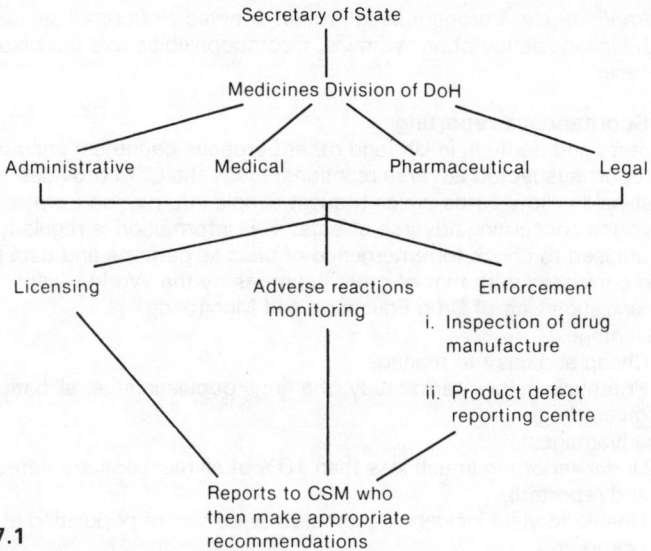

Secretary of State

Medicines Division of DoH

Administrative   Medical   Pharmaceutical   Legal

Licensing   Adverse reactions monitoring   Enforcement

i. Inspection of drug manufacture

ii. Product defect reporting centre

Reports to CSM who then make appropriate recommendations

Fig. 7.1

Adverse reaction monitoring

Continued surveillance is required even after grant of a product licence since on release of a drug only common, short-term and obvious adverse effects will have been discovered because at most only 2000–5000 individuals will have received the drug. Thus detection of events with incidence <1 in 1000 unlikely.

Number of patients required to detect 1, 2, or 3 cases of an adverse reaction (assuming no 'background' incidence):

Incidence of adverse reaction	No. of patients required to detect		
	1 case	2 cases	3 cases
1 in 200	600	960	1 300
1 in 2000	6 000	9 600	13 000
1 in 10 000	30 000	48 000	65 000

Mechanisms for discovery of adverse effects include:

1. Formal clinical trials

Advantages:
a. Close observation of individual patients.
b. Allows assessment of incidence of effects.
Disadvantages:
a. Few patients enrolled.
b. Main aim usually to assess efficacy not side effects.
c. Patients may be atypical of general clinical practice.
d. Short period of observation (long-term trials expensive and difficult to organise).

Example of use: Coronary Drug Project showed clofibrate associated with high incidence of arrhythmias, thrombophlebitis and gall bladder disease.

2. Spontaneous reporting

Doctors and dentists in UK (and other European countries) encouraged to report suspected adverse reactions. In UK the CSM provides post-paid yellow cards which request simple information from clinicians concerning adverse effects. This information is regularly scrutinised to check for emergence of unusual patterns and data is also correlated with that of other countries by the World Health Organization Unit of Drug Education and Monitoring.

Advantages:
a. Cheap and easy to manage.
b. Potentially a long-term study of a huge population (i.e. all patients given drug).

Disadvantages:
a. Under-reporting (much less than 10% of all reactions are detected and reported).
b. Unable to yield incidence estimates since size of population at risk unknown.
c. Not a uniformly sampled population and data may be unrepresentative. Liable to 'band-wagon' effects, i.e. well-known effects over-reported, but unsuspected or bizarre events go unrecorded.
d. Not been very successful in reporting previously unsuspected effects.

Example of use: Withdrawal of ibufenac from UK after reports of liver damage.

3. Vital statistics

Review of epidemiological data from death certificates, hospital discharge summaries etc. to look for unexpected trends or effects.

Advantages:
a. Potentially a large scale chronic study of drug effects.
b. Could be relatively cheap.
c. Unbiased by pre-conceived hypotheses.

Disadvantages:
a. Most of the necessary data (like drug exposure) is not presently accessible.
b. Slow and cumbersome in present practice.
c. Does not establish causality of relationship.

Example of use: Linkage of sudden death with use of isoprenaline bronchodilator aerosol inhalation.

4. Case control studies

Drug history of patients with disease compared to that of control population.

Advantage:
a. Easier and cheaper than following the necessarily much larger population only some of whom will develop reaction.
Disadvantages:
a. Difficult in practice because danger of bias in selection of control due to a *priori* hypothesis.
b. Gives relative risk but not an incidence of effects.
c. Does not establish causal effect of drug.
Example of use: Association of lincomycin exposure with pseudomembranous colitis.

5. Monitored release and post-marketing surveillance

Aim is to follow a large cohort (say 10 000) patients given new drug for long period (> 1 year). Use mainly confined to new drugs but potentially also for older drugs especially in high risk groups, e.g. old, renal failure.
Advantages:
a. Acute and chronic effects monitored.
b. Cheaper than a long-term clinical trial.
c. Gives assessment of incidence.
Disadvantages:
a. Difficult to maintain integrity of patient group.
b. Lacks a control group for comparison since in long-term studies other factors, e.g. nutrition, radiation levels, may also change.

6. Intensive monitoring

Can be of variable intensity from analysis of hospital records (e.g. Aberdeen–Dundee Monitoring system) to use of special wards with personnel exclusively for monitoring drug effects and use complementary to usual management team (e.g. Boston Collaborative Drug Surveillance Program). Data collected is stored on computer and regularly examined for trends and associations.
Advantages:
a. Not *a priori* hypothesis therefore no bias.
b. Can detect unexpected effects.
c. All possible information stored so incidence, associated factors, e.g. age, sex, electrolyte status, can be extracted.
Disadvantages:
a. Expensive.
b. Relatively small scale studies so only common reactions will be detected.
c. Only acute effects monitored.
d. Patient sample restricted and could be unrepresentative.
Example of use: Link of ethacrynic acid with gastrointestinal bleeding especially when given i.v. to females, with high blood urea who had previously received heparin.

General comments
1. All drugs are dangerous — in general, drugs without side-effects are also without any effects, good or bad.
2. For most drugs there is insufficient information to provide a risk–benefit analysis. Ask advice from senior doctors if in doubt and build up your experience by getting to know a restricted range of drugs.
3. Drugs should only be used when there are clear indications and no alternatives.
4. Always take a drug history.
5. Restrict the number of drugs prescribed to the minimum.
6. Regularly review the need for chronic medication.
7. Clearly record what drugs are prescribed, their dose and frequency for the benefit of others who may look after the patient.
8. Exercise special care in the use of certain groups of drugs (see earlier) and in the young, the elderly, and patients with organ impairment.
9. Contribute to knowledge of drugs by reporting on a yellow card cases where an adverse effect occurs on drug therapy.
10. Keep the patient informed about the treatment and what he may expect from it.

8. Drugs for psychiatric and CNS disease

ANTIDEPRESSANTS

Older tricyclics (e.g. amitriptyline; dothiepin)
Tetracyclic and other structures (e.g. mianserin; viloxazine; iprindole)
5HT uptake blockers: mixed (e.g. trazodone; lofepramine)
selective (e.g. fluvoxamine; fluoxetine)
Monoamine oxidase inhibitors (e.g. phenelzine)
Thioxanthines (e.g. flupenthixol)

Other agents
Prophylactic (e.g. lithium; carbamazepine)
Selegiline with low tyramine diet for atypical depression

Indications for tricyclic and related antidepressants
Endogenous depression — usually good response
Neurotic depressive syndromes — usually poor response
Schizo-affective syndromes — some patients respond well
Phobic anxiety
Depression in obsessive compulsive disorders $\left\{ \begin{array}{l} \text{clomipramine or} \\ \text{imipramine are} \\ \text{used} \end{array} \right.$

Atypical facial pain — usually good response
Enuresis — imipramine used, not very successful

General properties of tricyclic antidepressants
1. *Mode of action*
   block of neuronal uptake$_1$ of NA, 5HT or dopamine (tertiary amines mainly block uptake of 5HT, secondary mainly NA)
2. *Pharmacological*
   anticholinergic (especially tertiary amines)
   sympathomimetic (e.g. produce cardiac arrhythmias)
   epileptogenic
3. *Pharmacokinetic*
   well absorbed but variable and sometimes extensive 1st pass metabolism

some metabolites are active
relatively long $T_{1/2}$ but much individual variation
large volume of distribution (e.g. imipramine V_d = 28–61 l/kg)
high plasma protein binding.

4. *Response*
   a. Optimal clinical response may occur within a range of plasma concentrations.
   b. Clinical response usually delayed for 1–3 weeks.

5. *A. Common toxic effects*
   a. *Anticholinergic*: dry mouth, bad taste, blurred vision, glaucoma aggravated, hesitancy of micturition, impotence, delayed orgasm, constipation.
   b. *Cardiovascular*: postural hypotension (weak α-adrenergic blockers), palpitations. Overdose: supraventricular tachycardia, ventricular tachycardia, A-V block, bundle branch block, prolonged PR, QRS, QT intervals, T wave flattening, ST depression.
   c. *CNS*: tremor, sedation (especially tertiary amines), headache, heavy sleep, disturbed sleep, restlessness, choreiform movements, myoclonus, paraesthesiae, driving accidents, withdrawal syndrome (anxiety, restlessness, insomnia, anorexia).
   d. *Alimentary*: increased appetite, weight gain, anticholinergic effects.

   B. Uncommon toxic effects (important but rare effects italicised)
   a. *Anticholinergic*: paralytic ileus, oesophageal reflux, *acute retention*.
   b. *Cardiovascular: sudden death due to ventricular fibrillation*, cardiomyopathy, hypertension, atrial fibrillation, quinidine-like activity.
   c. *CNS: epileptic seizures* (may alter drug requirement of known epileptics), nightmares, acute confusional psychosis, hypomania.
   d. *Alimentary*: cholestatic jaundice.
   e. *Allergic*: cholestatic jaundice, urticaria, cutaneous vasculitis, angioedema, photosensitivity dermatitis.

   C. Contraindications
   a. recent myocardial infarction; arrhythmias; cardiomyopathy
   b. pregnancy
   c. prostatic hypertrophy
   d. glaucoma
   e. epilepsy
   f. liver failure
   g. renal failure.

   D. Drug interactions
   a. increased sedation with central depressants including alcohol
   b. MAOI: hypertension, hyperpyrexia, excitement, coma, cerebral haemorrhage, death

Table 3(a) Tricyclic antidepressants — iminodibenzyls

Drug	Amine structure	Action (all block NA and 5HT uptake)	Pharmacokinetics	Special clinical features
Imipramine	Tertiary	Equally powerful inhibition of NA and 5HT uptake	$T_{1/2}$ = 4–8 h. Main metabolite is active — desipramine ($T_{1/2}$ = 12–25 h)	Dose 25–300 mg o.n. Little or no sedation. Can cause insomnia. Powerful anticholinergic
Desipramine (= desmethylimipramine = DMI)	Secondary	Very powerful inhibitor of NA uptake. Little or no action on 5HT	$T_{1/2}$ = 12–25 h	Dose 25–300 mg o.n. Minimal sedation. Minimal anticholinergic
Trimipramine	Tertiary	Powerful inhibition of 5HT uptake. Some effect on NA and dopamine uptake. Demethyl metabolite mainly acts on NA uptake	Demethyl metabolite is active	Dose 50–150 mg o.n. Very sedating. Moderate anticholinergic
Clomipramine	Tertiary	Powerful inhibition of 5HT uptake	Dose dependent kinetics. Steady state attained at 7 days. Active demethyl metabolite (steady state at 14 days). After a single dose detected in blood for 48 hours and urine for 7 days	Dose 10–150 mg o.n. Sedating. Postural hypotension

Table 3(b) Tricyclic antidepressants — dibenzocycloheptenes

Drug	Amine structure	Action (all block NA and 5HT uptake)	Pharmacokinetics	Special clinical features
Amitriptyline	Tertiary	Powerful blockade of 5HT uptake. Some action on NA uptake	$T_{1/2}$ = 8–20 h. Active metabolite is nortriptyline ($T_{1/2}$ = 18–93 h)	Dose 25–150 mg o.n. Strongly sedating. Powerful anticholinergic
Nortriptyline	Secondary	Powerful blockade of NA uptake. Some action on 5HT uptake	$T_{1/2}$ = 18–93 h	Dose 25–150 mg o.n. Less sedating than amitriptyline. Weak anticholinergic
Protriptyline	Secondary		$T_{1/2}$ = 54–198 h	Dose 15–60 mg o.n. Less sedation, may be stimulant. Moderately anticholinergic
Butriptyline	Tertiary	Weak inhibitor of NA and 5HT uptake	$T_{1/2}$ = 65–135 h (mainly metabolites). Much first pass metabolism	Dose 25–50 mg 8 hourly

Table 3(c) Tricyclic antidepressants — anxiolytic

Drug	Pharmacokinetics	Special clinical features
Doxepin	$T\frac{1}{2}$ = 8–20 h. Active metabolite — desmethyldoxepin ($T\frac{1}{2}$ = 33–81 h). Extensive (55–87%) first pass metabolism, but well absorbed from intestine	Least adverse effects on CVS of tricyclics. Optimal antidepressant at plasma levels of desmethyldoxepin above 20 ng/ml
Dothiepin	$T\frac{1}{2}$ = 46–56 h	Both these drugs are less powerful antidepressants than amitriptyline, but have a lower incidence of anticholinergic toxic effects. Also have benzodiazepine-like anxiolytic actions

   c. lithium: increased tremor
   d. phenothiazines: increase sedation, hypotension, anticholinergic effects and cardiac arrhythmias
   e. stimulants (e.g. amphetamines): excitement, hypertension, hyperpyrexia, cardiac arrhythmias
   f. increased anticholinergic effects with anticholinergics
   g. abolition of hypotensive action of clonidine and adrenergic neurone blockers (e.g. debrisoquine, bethanidine)
   h. possible rise in blood pressure with directly acting sympathomimetics
   i. tricyclic plasma levels lowered by inducing agents (e.g. barbiturates).

Point about newer antidepressants (lofepramine, mianserin, trazodone, viloxazine):
No claim for greater potency over tricyclics or MAOI. Less cardiotoxic and less anticholinergic than older tricyclics.

Selective inhibitors of 5HT uptake
Fluvoxamine, fluoxetine, sertraline and paroxetine are antidepressive. Fluoxetine and sertraline have been tried in prophylaxis.
    All these 5HT uptake blockers are not sedating, but can cause nausea, tremor, sexual dysfunction and dizziness. Rarely fluoxetine is associated with a fatal vasculitis.

MONOAMINE OXIDASE INHIBITORS

General properties
Inhibit MAO and some other oxidases.
Increased intracerebral and peripheral neural stores of amines

(including NA). Amine stores discharged by indirectly acting sympathomimetics. Increased α stimulation of the vasomotor centre which results in reflex hypotension. Clinical response delayed up to 2–6 weeks. MAO is irreversibly inhibited so effects continue for about 2 weeks after stopping treatment.
Phenelzine (Nardil) most widely used.

Uses
1. Some neurotic depressive syndromes.
2. Endogenous depression which has failed to respond to tricyclic antidepressants.
3. Some forms of atypical facial pain.
4. Anxiety with depression; phobic anxiety, obsessive — compulsive disorders.

Toxic effects
1. Food interactions.
2. Drug interactions.
3. *NS*: headaches, aggravation of migraine, drowsiness. *Autonomic effects*: dry mouth, hesitancy of micturition, postural hypotension.
4. Alimentary: anorexia, vomiting, hepatocellular damage.

Food interactions
Foods containing amines (which can cause a hypertensive reaction): cheeses, meat and yeast extracts (e.g. Marmite), some wines (e.g. Chianti), and beers (e.g. Worthington, Bass), game, banana skins*, broad bean pods, pickled herrings, green figs, roe products.

Drug interactions
1. *Hypertensive reactions*
   a. indirectly acting sympathomimetics (e.g. amphetamines, ephedrine, phenylethylamine, metaraminol and cocaine)
   b. less hypertensive reactions from directly acting sympathomimetics (e.g. adrenaline, noradrenaline, phenylephrine)
   c. levodopa
   d. tricyclics (but such very dangerous combinations used by specialists in small doses for refractory depression).
2. *Effects potentiated of* opioids and hypnotics.
3. *Excitement or confusion* with anticholinergic, antiparkinsonian drugs (e.g. benztropine).

LITHIUM

Uses
Established
1. Acute mania (improvement or remission in 70–80% patients).

---

*Mysteriously, banana skins are said to be used in the manufacture of some wines.

Table 4 Antidepressants developed after older tricyclics

Drug	Structure	Mode of action	Special features
Mianserin	True tetracyclic	Inhibition of prejunctional (α_2) noradrenergic receptors. Some post-synaptic blockade of 5HT	Sedating, not sympathomimetic, not anticholinergic. 'Safe' in overdose. Hypotension. $T\frac{1}{2}$ = 15 h. Agranulocytosis rare
Maprotilene	Tricyclic with additional methylene bridge, i.e. tetracyclic	Inhibition reuptake NA. Some inhibition reuptake 5HT	Less sympathomimetic and anticholinergic than tricyclics. Epileptogenic. $T\frac{1}{2}$ = 48 h
Trazodone	Not tricyclic	Blocks 5HT uptake	Sedating and anxiolytic. Weakly anticholinergic. 'Safe' in overdose $T\frac{1}{2}$ = 5 h. Priapism rare
Lofepramine	Tricyclic	Metabolite blocks NA and 5HT reuptake	40% converted to desipramine. Safer in overdose, less sedation and less anticholinergic than amitriptyline
Amoxapine	Related to neuroleptic loxapine	Blocks NA and 5HT uptake. Also blocks DA receptors	Mildly anticholinergic and sedating. Can cause tardive dyskinesias and fits
Viloxazine	Bicyclic	Blocks NA uptake	Little sedation but causes nausea

2. Prophylactic in manic-depressive illness (cyclothymia).
3. Prophylactic in recurrent unipolar affective illness (depression or mania). As effective as tricyclics.
4. *Not yet established* in cluster headaches.

Pharmacokinetics
Readily absorbed from gut — peak plasma levels at 3–5 hours.
$T\frac{1}{2}$ = 18–20 h (up to 36 h in elderly) — becomes longer (50 + h) with prolonged therapy.

Not bound to plasma proteins.
Renal elimination: readily filtered at glomerulus; 75% reabsorbed in proximal tubules in competition with Na^+; no distal reabsorption. Elimination accelerated by sodium; impaired by sodium deficiency and by diuretics because of competitive effects in proximal tubule.

Administration
Response starts after 2–4 weeks in prophylaxis and 10 days in hypomania. Full benefit in 6–12 months.

Therapeutic plasma levels
Mania 0.4–1.0 mmol/l 12 h after dose. Prophylaxis 0.4–0.8 mmol/l 12 h after dose. Check levels every 3 months.

Toxic effects
Dose dependent
0.8–1.2 mmol/l: mild tremor
1.5–3 mmol/l: tremor, ataxia, weakness, drowsiness, thirst, diarrhoea
3–5 mmol/l: severe tremor, confusion, spasticity, convulsions, dehydration, coma, death
Chronic renal damage related to chronic dosage. Consider limiting treatment to 3–5 years only.

Dose independent
1. Goitre, hypothyroidism (10%), hyperthyroidism (rare).
2. Nephrogenic diabetes insipidus (? Li inhibits ADH stimulation of adenyl cyclase), hyperaldosteronism.
3. Reversible ECG changes; cardiac arrhythmias.
4. Loss of bone calcium.
5. Weight gain.

Drug interactions
1. Thiazides, loop diuretics enhance lithium retention and toxicity because of sodium depletion.
2. Tardive dyskinesias and other extrapyramidal syndromes due to neuroleptics made commoner. (Lithium can be used with tricyclics and MAOI).
3. Earlier lithium plasma peak with metoclopramide.
4. Delayed lithium plasma peak with anticholinergics.

Pregnancy
1. ?Increased incidence of cardiovascular malformations particularly if given in first trimester.
2. Breast feeding contraindicated — Li excreted in milk.

NEUROLEPTICS (ANTIPSYCHOTIC DRUGS)
1. Reduce stimulation of dopamine receptors usually by D_2 receptor blockade.

2. Effective in excited psychotic states, hallucinations and delirium. Clinical potency correlates well with ability to block central dopamine receptors.

Main actions of phenothiazine neuroleptics
1. Central
Anti-hallucinatory and anti-psychotic
Reduction in emotional responsiveness (ataractic state)
Sedation and reduction in attention span wth slower learning
Antiemetic, anti-hiccough
Produces extrapyramidal syndromes, but can reduce chorea
Aggravation of epilepsy
Hypothalamic inhibition: reduced sympathetic outflow
                            loss of temperature control
                            increased prolactin release

2. Peripheral
α-adrenoceptor blockade
Anticholinergic
Quinidine-like action on heart.

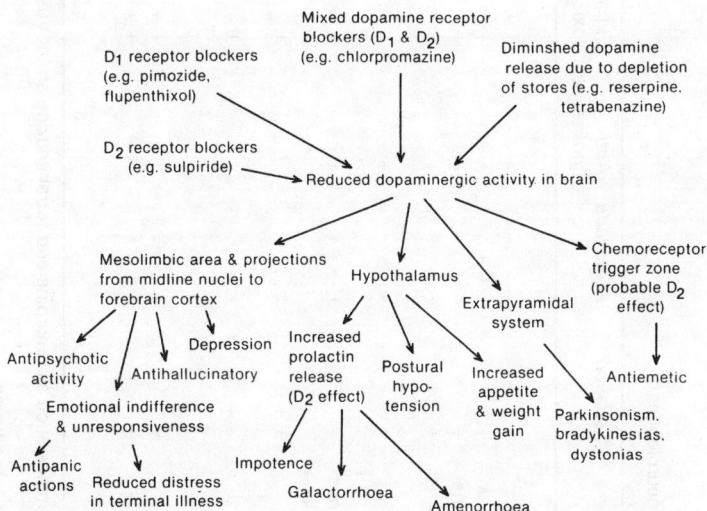

Mixed dopamine receptor blockers (D_1 & D_2) (e.g. chlorpromazine)

D_1 receptor blockers (e.g. pimozide, flupenthixol)

Diminshed dopamine release due to depletion of stores (e.g. reserpine. tetrabenazine)

D_2 receptor blockers (e.g. sulpiride) → Reduced dopaminergic activity in brain

Mesolimbic area & projections from midline nuclei to forebrain cortex

Hypothalamus

Chemoreceptor trigger zone (probable D_2 effect)

Extrapyramidal system

Antipsychotic activity

Depression

Antihallucinatory

Increased prolactin release (D_2 effect)

Postural hypotension

Increased appetite & weight gain

Antiemetic

Emotional indifference & unresponsiveness

Parkinsonism. bradykinesias. dystonias

Antipanic actions

Reduced distress in terminal illness

Impotence

Galactorrhoea

Amenorrhoea

(Dopamine D_1 receptors: adenyl cyclase linked (like β receptors)
Dopamine D_2 receptors: not linked with adenyl cyclase)

Fig. 8.1 Role of dopamine in actions of neuroleptics

Toxicity of the phenothiazine neuroleptics
1. Postural hypotension.

Table 5 Main types of neuroleptics

Group	Sedation	α-blockade	Anti-cholinergic	Extra pyramidal toxicity	Special features
1. Phenothiazines					
a. aliphatic side chains	+ + +	+ +	+ +	+ +	Antiemetic
b. piperidine side chains	+ + +	+ + +	+ + +	+ +	Not antiemetic
c. piperazine side chains	+	+	+	+ + +	Some are stimulant Powerfully antiemetic
2. Butyrophenones	+	+	+	+ + +	Similar to piperazine phenothiazines Powerfully antiemetic
3. Thioxanthines e.g. flupenthixol	+ → + + +	+ +	+ +	+ +	Antidepressant
4. Diphenylbutylpiperidines e.g. pimozide; fluspirilene	+	± → +	±	±	Long acting after oral administration Powerful antipsychotic activity
5. Dihydroindoles e.g. oxypertine	+ +	±		+	
6. Dibenzodiazepines e.g. clozapine	+ +	+ +	+ +	±	For resistant schizophrenia. Little neurological toxicity, but may be toxic to marrow. Regular blood counts essential
7. Benzamides	+ +	+ +	+ +	+ +	Causes neurological toxicity
8. Loxapine	+ +	+ +	+ +	+ +	Can cause dermatitis, seborrhoea, pruritus and photosensitivity, nausea, headache

(Depletors of cerebral amines such as reserpine and tetrabenazine are not usually used as neuroleptics as they are prone to produce depression)
± = very little   + + = moderate
+ = mild   + + + = considerable

2. Dry mouth, nasal stuffiness, failure of ejaculation, constipation, urinary retention, blurred vision.
3. Sedation, drowsiness, confusion, depression, emotional inertia.
4. Convulsions.
5. Tremor, Parkinsonism, dystonia, dyskinesia, akathisia (motor restlessness), tardive dyskinesias.
6. Cholestatic jaundice (2–4% of patients on chlorpromazine, especially during 2nd–4th week of treatment) — often associated with eosinophilia.
7. Corneal and lens opacities, pigmentary retinopathy.
8. Light sensitivity dermatitis and pigmentation, urticaria, oedema, maculopapular and petechial rashes.
9. Raised cholesterol, impaired glucose tolerance.
10. Leucopenia, thrombocytopenia (both very rare).
11. Cardiac arrhythmias, cardiac arrest.
12. Oligomenorrhoea, amenorrhoea, gynaecomastia, galactorrhoea.
13. Malignant syndrome (coma, autonomic disturbances).

Drug interactions with the phenothiazines
1. Anticholinergic effects on gastrointestinal tract affect absorption of paracetamol, levodopa, digoxin, lithium.
2. Alcohol potentiates sedation.
3. Effects of hypnotics and anxiolytics potentiated.
4. Sedative, respiratory depressant and 'cortical' effects of narcotic analgesics potentiated.
5. Potentiation of hypotensive drugs.

Clinical uses of phenothiazines
Psychiatry
— schizophrenia
— hypomania
— delirium
— drug withdrawal (but not alcohol and hypnotics)
— panic attacks
α-blockade
— shock
— hypertension — reactions with MAOI
Terminal illness
Antiemetic, antihiccough, Ménière's disease
Surgery
— premedication
— hypothermic techniques
— neuroleptanalgesia.

Depot neuroleptics
Fluphenazine decanoate, fluphenazine enanthate and flupenthixol injected i.m. every 2–4 weeks.

Table 5a Individual neuroleptic drugs

Drug	Pharmacokinetics	Special uses apart from in psychoses
1. Phenothiazines		
a. Aliphatic side chain		
Chlorpromazine	$T\frac{1}{2}$ = 2–24 h. V_d = 22 1/kg 30% bioavailability after oral administration. Incompletely absorbed. Completely absorbed after i.m. injection. 70 metabolites. Cpz and 7-OH are active, Cpz sulphoxide is inactive.	Antiemetic, sedation in elderly and violent patients without causing stupor. Narcotic withdrawal. Anti-hiccough.
Promazine		Not sufficiently active to be used in psychosis but useful tranquilliser — especially in elderly.
b. Piperidine side chain		
Thioridazine	$T\frac{1}{2}$ = 10–36 h. Active metabolite is mesoridazine. Prolonged $T\frac{1}{2}$ in elderly. Metabolism slowed during sleep.	Useful for agitated old patients — less extrapyramidal effects. More postural hypotension.
c. Piperazine side chain		
Trifluoperazine		Tranquilliser in behavioural disturbance and psychoneuroses. Antiemetic.
Prochlorperazine		Ménière's disease. Antiemetic
Perphenazine	$T\frac{1}{2}$ = 9 h	Antiemetic. Anti-hiccough
2. Butyrophenones		
Haloperidol	$T\frac{1}{2}$ = 12–38 h. Well absorbed, but 60% bioavailability. Metabolised to inactive products. 1st order elimination. Metabolism slowed during sleep.	Anaesthetic premed, withdrawal of narcotics, Gilles de la Tourette syndrome. Tranquillisation in acute behavioural disturbances, especially mania.
Benperidol		Deviant and antisocial sexual behaviour.
Droperidol		Anaesthetic premed, antiemetic, given with narcotic for neuroleptanalgesia.
Trifluoperidol		Tranquillisation in acute behavioural disturbances, especially mania.

An initial test dose is usually given to determine susceptibility to extrapyramidal reactions. May need concurrent anti-Parkinsonian drugs but dosage reduction may be more effective in minimising these reactions with long-term therapy.

Advantages
1. Avoids high GI and hepatic first-pass metabolism giving reliable absorption.
2. Oily ester slowly hydrolysed and absorbed from muscle giving constant blood levels.
3. No compliance problem.

Management of acutely disturbed patients
1. Establish cause
   — system failure? (brain disease, cardiac, respiratory, hepatic, renal failure)
   — infection?
   — drug-induced? e.g. alcohol
   — silent myocardial infarction?
   — nutritional?
   — pneumonia?
   — postoperative?
   — acute psychosis?
2. Provide stable comforting environment: side room with night lights; reassure; infrequent changes of nurses; enlist relatives and friends to be with patient.
3. Sedate only when necessary because masks physical signs. Use oral drugs (syrups useful) if possible (injections can be difficult to give and encourage paranoia).

ANXIOLYTIC DRUGS

Anxiolytic = a drug which ameliorates feelings of tension and anxiety. All hypnotics have anxiolytic actions and all anxiolytics have hypnotic properties.

Benzodiazepines
Powerfully anxiolytic drugs which act in the CNS by potentiating the action of the inhibitory transmitter, GABA, by facilitating specific benzodiazepine receptors which are associated with post-synaptic GABA receptors. Flumazenil can bind to these benzodiazepine receptors and block the sedative, psychomotor and subjective effects of diazepam. It terminates the action of these drugs and is used to help diagnosis of benzodiazepine overdose.

Actions
1. Anxiolytic; sedative (not analgesic, not antidepressive, not antipsychotic)

Table 6 Drug-induced extrapyramidal disorders

Syndrome	Mechanism	Causative drugs	Treatment
Parkinsonism: complete syndrome or single features: tremor, akinesia, rigidity, oculogyric crises	Blockade of extrapyramidal dopamine receptors or depletion of dopamine stores	Neuroleptics Reserpine Tetrabenazine Methyldopa (Metoclopramide — rarely)	Anticholinergic, e.g. benzhexol 5–15 mg orally daily (modest improvement)
Acute dystonic reactions: within 48 h of start of treatment abrupt onset of retrocollis, torticollis, facial grimacing, dysarthria, laboured breathing, involuntary movements, scoliosis, lordosis, opisthotonus, dystonic gait. Children and adolescents most susceptible	? Increase in transmitter turnover	Neuroleptics Metoclopramide Domperidone Levodopa	i.v. diazepam 5–20 mg i.v. benztropine 2 mg
Akathisia: motor restlessness after days, weeks or months of treatment	Overstimulation or increased sensitivity of central dopamine receptors	Neuroleptics Levodopa	Reduction in drug therapy, drug holiday, benzodiazepines. But akathisia may resolve spontaneously
Chronic tardive dyskinesias: oro-facial chewing and sucking movements, accompanied by distal limb chorea and dystonia of trunk. 15% of patients treated with neuroleptics for more than 2 years develop this. Often persists or worsens on stopping drug. Stop during sleep, reduced by distraction, worsened by emotion	Structural injury in extrapyramidal system. Denervation hypersensitivity with increase in the number of dopamine receptors in affected neurones	Neuroleptics Lithium Metoclopramide Domperidone	No known satisfactory treatment. Neuroleptics continued. Perhaps some benefit from calcium antagonists, α-tocopherol, pimozide or thiopropazate; reserpine or tetrabenazine (depletes amines); lithium (? decreases amine release); choline or lecithin (?increases acetylcholine). Worsened with anticholinergics

2. Muscle relaxant
3. Anticonvulsant
4. Increase appetite
5. Anterograde amnesia (high blood levels).

Adverse effects
1. CNS
   a. *mainly dose dependent*: sedation, fatigue, somnolence, muscle weakness, diplopia, blurring of vision, ataxia, dysarthria, incoordination, apathy, impaired memory, prolonged reaction time (and traffic accidents)
   b. *rare paradoxical effects*: excitement, rage
   c. *other rare effects*: Korsakoff-type amnesic syndrome, hypnagogic hallucinations.
2. Relatively little CVS and respiratory depression (but large doses lethal if taken with other central depressants or in lung disease). Apnoea if large i.v. dose given rapidly.
3. Allergy uncommon.
4. Dependence (physical and psychic): withdrawal state (1–10 days delay) lasts many weeks. Characterised by insomnia, anxiety, dyspepsia, depression, muscular pains, hypersensitivity to touch, sound and light, fits.
5. Drug interactions: potentiation by other CNS depressants; very weak inducer.
6. Local:
   a. intravenous diazepam: pain, thrombophlebitis
   b. intra-arterial: spasm, pain, ischaemia, gangrene.

Diazemuls is a lipid suspension of diazepam for i.v. injection with reduced tendency to produce thrombophlebitis.

Midazolam: a shorter acting intravenous benzodiazepine used for endoscopy (see Table 7).

Metabolic interrelationships of some benzodiazepines (Fig. 8.2)

Benzodiazepine pharmacokinetics
A useful classification of benzodiazepines subdivides according to ranges of half-life (see Table 7).

Many form active metabolites with long $T½$. Therapeutic effect of several is due to same metabolite and so these may not offer real alternatives.

Buspirone is an anxiolytic which does not act via benzodiazepine receptors. It binds to $5HT_{1A}$ receptors, and is a partial serotoninergic agonist.

Half-life 2–11 h, but action may be delayed for up to 4 weeks. Buspirone is less sedative than benzodiazepines, but headache, nausea and giddiness are more common. Dependence has not yet been demonstrated.

Table 7 Benzodiazepines

Drug	Active metabolites	$T_{1/2}$ (h) of parent compound	Special features
Longer acting			
Diazepam	Desmethyldiazepam ($T_{1/2}$ 36–200 h) Oxazepam	20–50	General 'all purpose' benzodiazepine but also useful i.v. in status epilepticus. i.m. injection poorly absorbed
Chlordiazepoxide	Desmethylchlordiazepoxide Desmethyldiazepam Oxazepam	3–30	i.m. injection poorly absorbed (precipitates at injection site)
Clorazepate	Desmethyldiazepam Oxazepam	30–60	Parent drug completely metabolised to desmethyl diazepam (i.e. is a prodrug)
Nitrazepam	None	24	Hypnotic use but also anticonvulsant
Flurazepam	Desalkylflurazepam ($T_{1/2}$ = 40–250 h) Hydroxethylflurazepam	2	Hypnotic
Medazepam	Desmethylmedazepam Desmethyldiazepam	Probably about 24 h	
Clobazam	N-desmethyl-clobazam	24	Claimed to produce no psychomotor impairment. Less hypnotic and muscle relaxant effects than diazepam
Clonazepam	None	30	Mainly used as an anticonvulsant
Shorter acting with no active metabolites			
Oxazepam	None	5–20	
Lorazepam	None	10–20	Useful i.v. in status epilepticus. Well absorbed by i.m. injection — thus useful in delirium tremens
Temazepam	None	5–20	
Ultra-short acting			
Triazolam	Hydroxytriazolam	2–4	Used only as hypnotic Psychotic reactions have been reported
Midazolam	Hydroxymidazolam ($T_{1/2}$ 1–1 1/2 h)		Used i.v. for profound psychosedation, e.g. endoscopy

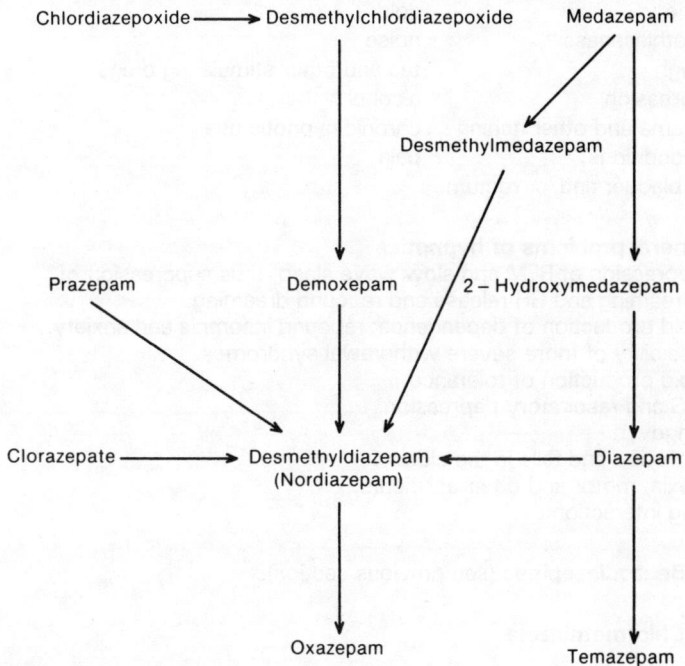

Chlordiazepoxide ⟶ Desmethylchlordiazepoxide   Medazepam

Desmethylmedazepam

Prazepam   Demoxepam   2 – Hydroxymedazepam

Clorazepate ⟶ Desmethyldiazepam ⟵ Diazepam
                (Nordiazepam)

Oxazepam   Temazepam

Fig. 8.2

Treatment of chronic anxiety

1. Drugs are generally avoided in chronic anxiety.
2. Non drug treatment includes simple psychotherapy, relaxation training, cognitive therapy and behaviour therapy.
3. Drugs — rarely used
    a. benzodiazepines — not for prolonged use
    b. MAOI — for phobic anxiety and panic attacks
    c. tricyclics for generalised anxiety, phobias and panic attacks — may initially increase restlessness
    d. β-blockers — for tremor and palpitations
    e. buspirone — undergoing assessment.

HYPNOTICS

Greatly over-prescribed (over 45s: 45% women and 15% men take them!) Commonest reason for 'insomnia' is reduced physiological need with age. Also exclude common primary causes of insomnia:

anxiety	cold
breathlessness	noise
cough	tea and other stimulating drugs
depression	alcohol
eczema and other itching conditions	chronic hypnotic use
	pain
full bladder and/or rectum	

General problems of hypnotics
Suppression of REM and slow wave sleep, thus suppression of
    dreaming and GH release and rebound dreaming.
Rapid production of dependence; rebound insomnia and anxiety.
Possibility of more severe withdrawal syndromes.
Rapid production of tolerance.
CVS and respiratory depression.
Hangover.
Confusion and falls in the elderly.
Ataxia, motor and other accidents.
Drug interactions.

1. Benzodiazepines (see previous section).

2. Chlormethiazole

Pharmacokinetics
$T_{1/2} = 1$ h; time to peak = 1 h; Extensive (85%) first pass metabolism;
(bioavailability increased to nearly 100% in liver disease).

Toxicity
1. Nasal, conjunctival and bronchial discomfort
2. Gastric irritation
3. Respiratory and CVS depression
4. 2% solution IV can cause thrombophlebitis and haemolysis
5. Dependence.

Uses
1. Hypnotic (especially in elderly)
2. Acute withdrawal from alcohol, barbiturates, narcotic analgesics
3. i.v. in status epilepticus.

3. Zopiclone
A non-benzodiazepine hypnotic but with similar toxicity. Causes
metallic taste. Half-life 5-6 h; inactive metabolites.
    After continuous use, withdrawal is accompanied by insomnia and
anxiety.

4. Chloral

Pharmacokinetics
Well absorbed, rapidly metabolised (reduced) to more active trichlorethanol ($T\frac{1}{2}$ = 8 h).

Toxicity
1. Respiratory and CVS depression
2. Gastric irritation
3. Rashes: erythematous, scarlatiniform, urticarial, scaling
4. Jaundice
5. Proteinuria
6. Interactions: alcohol ('Mickey Finn'), warfarin (see Chapter 6).

EPILEPSY

Before treating, ask:
1. Are the fits epileptic rather than another disorder (e.g. syncope, cardiac arrhythmia, sleep paralysis, hypoglycaemia, hyperventilation)?
2. Is the epilepsy secondary to a treatable condition (e.g. tumour)?
3. Are there treatable factors which precipitate the epilepsy (e.g. flashing light, hangover, hunger)?
4. Is there a significant risk of further fits if the patient is left untreated?

If treatment is decided on:
1. The type of epilepsy suggests a choice of drug (see Table below).
2. Initially a single drug at a time is tried — if necessary with the help of plasma levels.
3. Changes in drug treatment must not be sudden and gradual reduction of dose of one drug must accompany introduction of new drug.

NB Important to treat epilepsy as soon as possible: repeated seizure episodes worsen prognosis for control.

Main drugs in the treatment of epilepsy

Type of epilepsy	First line drugs
1. Generalised:	
Tonic clonic	Carbamazepine
	Sodium valproate
	Phenytoin
Simple absences	Sodium valproate and/or
	ethosuximide
Complex absences	Sodium valproate
	Clonazepam
	Clobazam

Type of epilepsy	*First line drugs*
Infantile spasms	ACTH or steroids
	Clonazepam
Myoclonic	Sodium valproate
epilepsy	Clonazepam

2. Partial and	Carbamazepine
secondarily	Sodium valproate
generalised	Phenytoin

Second line drugs for partial seizures

Vigabatrin	Clonazepam
Phenobarbitone	Primidone
Acetazolamide	Clobazam

Toxic effects of phenytoin
A. 1. *Nervous system*:
    cerebellar syndrome (ataxia, tremor, nystagmus, dysarthria)
    sedation
    depression, psychotic excitement, paranoia
    increased frequency of fits (rare consequence of high levels)
  2. *Immune disease and skin disorders*:
    allergic rashes
    acne
    systemic lupus erythematosus-like syndrome
  3. *Mesodermal changes*:
    coarsening of facial features
    gum hypertrophy (usually resolves on improved periodontal
      care)
    Dupuytren's contracture
    lymphadenopathy (very rarely lymphoma develops)
  4. *Haematological*:
    folate deficiency (common)
    megaloblastic anaemia (uncommon)
    aplastic anaemia (rare).
B. *Possible effects on fetus*: (but may be partly due to maternal
  fits)
    increased perinatal mortality
    raised frequency of cleft palate and hare lip
    microcephaly
    congenital heart disease.
C. *Drug interactions*:
  The following impair phenytoin metabolism:
    isoniazid
    chloramphenicol.

  The following accelerate phenytoin metabolism:
    ethanol
    carbamazepine.

Table 8 Drugs used in epilepsy

Drug	Effective plasma level	$T_{1/2}$	Pharmacokinetics	Toxicity
Ethosuximide	40–120 µg/ml	70 h adults 30 h children	Extensive metabolism to inactive products. Very little plasma protein binding	Non-toxic apart from mild giddiness, nausea and abdominal discomfort
Sodium valproate	40–80 µg/ml	7–10 h	Well absorbed. High plasma protein binding. Metabolites not yet identified, but effect persists beyond elimination from plasma	GI disturbances, enhancement of sedatives, temporary hair loss, false + ve ketone test in urine, weight gain, liver failure (rare), pancreatitis (rare)
Clonazepam	Not helpful	30 h	No active metabolites	Sedation, incoordination, hypotonia, dysphoria, paradoxical excitement
Clobazam	Not helpful	24 h	Desmethyl clobazam is active and has $T_{1/2}$ of over 2 days	As for clonazepam
Vigabatrin	Not helpful	5 h	Not an inducer. Not protein bound	Drowsiness, giddiness, confusion, psychotic reactions

Table 8 (continued)

Drug	Effective plasma level	$T_{1/2}$	Pharmacokinetics	Toxicity
Phenytoin	10–20 µg/ml (some patients well controlled with lower levels)	No single $T_{1/2}$ because zero order kinetics. Usually 12–120 h	Well absorbed, but bioavailability reduced if Ca^{++} given simultaneously. Great individual variation rate of metabolism	See text
Carbamazepine	4–10 µg/ml	Initially 25–60 h. 10 h on chronic administration, because of enzyme induction	Well absorbed. Partly metabolised to carbamazepine -10, 11 expoxide (active; $T_{1/2} = 2$ h). 75% plasma protein bound	Sedation, ataxia, giddiness, nystagmus, slurred speech, hyponatraemia and water intoxication. Enzyme inducer. Mild, reversible leucopenia common
Phenobarbitone	10–25 µg/ml	100 h adults 40 h children	Well absorbed. 50% bound to plasma proteins. Half is metabolised to inactive derivatives	Sedation, nystagmus, enzyme induction, paradoxical excitement, rebound fits on withdrawal, folate deficiency
Primidone		10 h (but long lived active metabolites)	2 active metabolites: phenobarbitone ($T_{1/2} = 100$ h) and phenylethylmalonamide ($T_{1/2} = 30$ h)	Sedation, nystagmus, enzyme induction, paradoxical excitement, rebound fits on withdrawal, folate deficiency

Phenytoin is an inducer and potentiates the metabolism of:
  oral contraceptives
  oral anticoagulants
  dexamethasone
  vitamin D
  folic acid.

Anticonvulsants in pregnancy

Congenital abnormalities in 7% of babies born to mothers taking anticonvulsants (cf. 2% in non-epileptic pregnancies).

Phenytoin associated with increased frequency of cleft lip and palate.

Valproate in the first trimester associated with 1–2% risk of spina bifida (i.e. 50 times the background rate).

Carbamazepine linked with craniofacial and other defects.

Febrile convulsions

Immediately. Many paediatricians admit a child to hospital who is having its first convulsion. All would admit a child with a fit lasting over 15 minutes or if there is no response to treatment or with evidence of intracranial disease.

Prolonged fits: intravenous or rectal diazepam. If fits persist then intravenous phenytoin or rectal paraldehyde. Lower fever with paracetamol and tepid sponging.

Further. Reassurance if a single fit. Reduce subsequent fevers. Some prescribe rectal diazepam to be given at the start of a subsequent fit.

Outlook. Most febrile seizures are brief and without sequelae. Very few of these children later develop epilepsy. Prophylaxis is rarely indicated.

Management of status epilepticus

Medical emergency, admit to intensive care unit.
1. Set up intravenous line, taking blood for levels of anticonvulsant drugs.
   Terminate fits as soon as possible with:
   i.v. benzodiazepines:
     diazepam 10 mg
     clonazepam 1 mg
     lorazepam 5 mg
   given over 2 minutes. Repeated if necessary. Alternatively i.v. chlormethiazole 0.8% (up to 500 mg in 6 h).
   If fits not controlled rapidly by above:
     i.v. thiopentone 150–750 mg
     intubation + muscle relaxant + artificial respiration.
2. Determine cause of status and treat if possible.
3. Recommence normal drug therapy as soon as possible. If patient not on drugs, a loading dose of phenytoin (15 mg/kg) via nasogastric tube.

PARKINSONISM

Drug-induced parkinsonism mediated via altered dopamine receptor activation.

Idiopathic and other forms of Parkinson's disease are due to degeneration of striatonigral pathway. Thus there are disturbances of acetycholine (excitatory) and dopamine (inhibitory) *receptor balance.*

Parkinsonism produced by chemicals:
1. blocking dopamine receptors (e.g. phenothiazines, butyrophenones)
2. depleting dopamine stores (e.g. reserpine)
3. interfering with dopamine synthesis (e.g. methyldopa)
4. selective neurotoxicity induced by methylphenyl-tetrahydropyridine (MPTP).

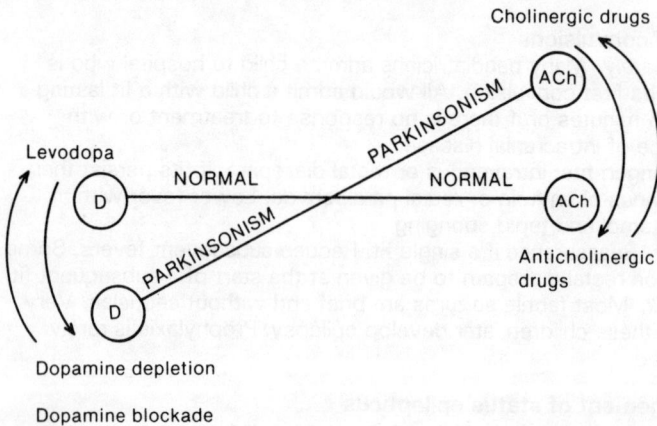

Fig. 8.3

Levodopa

Dopamine does not cross the blood–brain barrier but its precursor levodopa can and is metabolised to dopamine in situ by decarboxylase. Effective on all clinical features of Parkinson's disease.

Pharmacokinetics
About 40% of an oral dose absorbed. High protein diet reduces absorption by competition for the carrier by dietary amino acids. Most of absorbed drug is decarboxylated peripherally (mainly heart, blood vessels, gut, liver and kidneys). Peripheral decarboxylation enhanced by enzyme co-factor pyridoxine, which should be avoided in vitamin pills. $T_{1/2}$ is 1–5 h.

Levodopa is usually given with a decarboxylase inhibitor (e.g. carbidopa; benserazide). This raises the proportion of levodopa entering the brain.

Table 9 Drug induced movement disorders

Involuntary movement	Causative drugs	Clinical features	Onset after beginning therapy	Effect of drug withdrawal	Treatment
Parkinsonism	Phenothiazines Butyrophenones Reserpine Tetrabenazine Methyldopa (rare)	Dose dependent High incidence (~50%)	Gradual: several months	Reversible but slow to disappear	Anticholinergic drugs, levodopa not useful.
Tremor	β-agonists Lithium Tricyclic antidepressants	Dose dependent High incidence (~30%)	Rapid	Rapid reversal	None
Acute dystonia	Phenothiazines Butyrophenones Metoclopramide Diazoxide	Usually children or adolescents Low incidence (1–2%)	Rapid	Rapid reversal	Anticholinergic drugs Diazepam
Akathisia	Neuroleptics Methyldopa	High incidence (~30%)	Gradual: several months	Reversal over several days	Anticholinergic drugs
Tardive dyskinesias	Phenothiazines and other antipsychotics Metoclopramide Domperidone	High incidence (~30%) especially in elderly	Slow: several months or years	May worsen Persists in over 40%	No treatment known

Adverse effects
1. Gastrointestinal: nausea almost universal, usually subsides spontaneously at low doses but occasionally becomes dose-limiting.
2. Cardiovascular: mainly postural hypotension (due to central α-adrenergic receptor stimulation by noradrenaline, similar to action of clonidine, also peripheral inhibition of baroreceptor reflexes). Arrhythmias, mainly in patients with underlying heart disease so contraindicated in such patients and after myocardial infarction.
3. Involuntary movements — commonest dose-limiting reactions: facial grimacing, tongue movements, restlessness, jerking of the limbs.
4. Psychological: agitation, paranoia, confusion, depression, vivid nightmares may also limit dose.
5. Patients may become anxious about acidic urinary levodopa metabolites which stain clothing black or brown.
6. MAOI must be withdrawn 14 days before levodopa and should never be used concurrently since severe hypertension occurs.

Dopa decarboxylase inhibitors
Peripheral dopa decarboxylase inhibition reduces:
1. levodopa dose to produce optimum therapeutic benefit by 80%
2. incidence of nausea and vomiting
3. time to reach optimum dose
4. risk of cardiac arrhythmias and postural hypotension.
But involuntary movements and psychiatric side effects may be made more severe.

Two fixed combinations: levodopa plus benserazide (co-beneldopa) levodopa plus carbidopa (co-careldopa).

Problems of chronic levodopa treatment
1. Involuntary movements (chorea is commonest but also dystonia, myoclonus and ballistic movements). May occur at times related to dose:
   a. peak dose
   b. onset and end-of-dose
   c. nocturnal myoclonus
   d. early morning muscle cramps with dystonia.
2. Oscillation in performance:
   a. wearing-off effect — progressive reduction in duration of benefit from each dose.
   b. On–off effect — unpredictable swings from relative mobility to bradykinesia and hypotonia.
3. Toxic confusional states with nightmares and visual hallucinations.
4. ?Dementia is commoner.

Benefits
Bradykinesia and rigidity helped more than tremor.

Life expectancy is almost normal for patients who can tolerate levodopa.

Anticholinergic drugs
1. Block striatal muscarinic cholinergic receptors *but* also peripherally (causing glaucoma, urinary retention, constipation). Delirium, confusion and excitement may also result.
2. Rigidity and tremor respond best — akinesia unaffected (80% patients get 30% overall improvement).
3. Slowly increase from starting dose every 2–5 days until benefit or side effects occur.
4. May help Parkinsonism due to phenothiazines but never give prophylactically.
   Given i.v. for acute drug-induced dystonia and oculogyric crises.
NB Tardive dyskinesia is not improved, may worsen.

Amantadine
Developed as antiviral against Influenza A2, by chance found to improve Parkinsonism. Probably releases stored neuronal dopamine (acts similarly to amphetamine on adrenergic neurone).
   Akinesia, tremor and rigidity all respond but improvement considerably less (75–50%) than will levodopa and benefit may not be sustained. Can be used with levodopa or anticholinergics.
Drug-induced Parkinsonism refractory.

Adverse effects
Usually well tolerated but can cause restlessness, confusion, hallucinations, nightmares, livido reticularis and fits.

Bromocriptine
A dopamine agonist with similar actions to levodopa. Usually ineffective in patients not responsive to levodopa. Akinesia, rigidity and tremor all improve but may take 3 months to get optimum dose and response.
Duration of action prolonged (8–12 h) so less wearing-off effects. Psychiatric complications more common and dyskinesias less common than with levodopa. Can cause red painful extremities and pulmonary fibrosis.

Selegiline
Is an inhibitor of MAO–B commonly used with levodopa to reduce end of dose deterioration and decrease 'off' time in advanced disease. Hypertensive reactions do not occur with tyramine and other amines. Selegiline prolongs and intensifies the action of levodopa. However it causes insomnia and raises the risk of psychosis.
   Early treatment with selegiline may delay the need for levodopa and possibly slow the rate of progression of the disease. Life expectancy may be prolonged.

Lysuride
Lysuride is similar to bromocriptine. Can cause postural hypotension, expansion of pituitary tumours and aggravation of psychoses.

Pergolide
Pergolide is used with levodopa. Lysuride and pergolide are dopamine agonists which may be helpful in early or late disease but can cause psychoses.

DRUG TREATMENT OF MIGRAINE

ACUTE ATTACK

1. Antiemetics
   a. Metoclopramide antiemetic of choice in migraine — improves absorption of other drugs by accelerating gastric emptying 10 mg, tablet taken 10 minutes before other drugs (can also be given i.m.).
   b. Cyclizine tablet and injection.
   c. Triethylperazine tablet, injection and suppository.

2. Analgesics
Most attacks controlled by 900 mg aspirin or 1 g paracetamol or 125 mg flufenamic acid.

3. Anxiolytics
(e.g. diazepam 5 mg) May be helpful if given with analgesics. Useful if patient can sleep during an attack.

4. Ergotamine
Used only if analgesics plus metoclopramide have failed. Most patients with classical migraine will respond to analgesics plus metoclopramide plus ergotamine.
   Dose
(Older recommended doses are too high)
Dose per attack limited to
1–2 mg oral
or 1.08 mg inhaled
   Toxicity
1. Nausea, vomiting, headache, malaise.
2. Cold extremities, Raynaud's phenomena, claudication, paraesthesiae, gangrene (some of these vasospastic complications reversed by i.v. sodium nitroprusside).
3. Contraindicated in pregnancy.

5. Cyproheptadine
Antihistamine and anti-5-HT. Given orally 4–8 mg for acute attack or prophylaxis.

Toxicity
Sedation, anticholinergic, increased appetite.

6. Sumatriptan
Binds to 5HT 1A and 1D receptors. Effective in classical migraine and cluster headache. Acts by constricting cerebral arteries. Short half-life (2 h). Given by injection.

Toxicity
Includes pain on injection, tight feeling in chest, tingling, feeling of heat. Contraindicated in coronary artery disease and hemiplegic migraine.

PROPHYLAXIS

Not undertaken unless 2 attacks/month.
Not usually given to children.
Usually only necessary for months (not years).
1. β-blockers: propranolol 10–80 mg twice daily; atenolol 150 mg daily; effective in 50% patients.
   NB Never used with ergotamine because of increased risk of vascular disease.
2. Pizotifen (Sanomigran) A 5-HT antagonist.
   Toxicity: sedation, increased appetite and weight gain.
3. Low dose aspirin.
4. Antidepressants: imipramine or amitriptyline at night.
5. Methysergide: 5-HT antagonist and noradrenaline potentiator.
   Reduces 80% of headaches in 80% of patients. Rarely used because of toxicity: retroperitoneal and intrathoracic fibrosis (rare if dose kept low and used for not more than 6 consecutive months); GI disturbances; euphoria; hyperaesthesia; weight gain and oedema; constriction of large and small arteries.
NB Ergotamine tartrate should never be used in classical migraine as a prophylactic.
   Dihydroergotamine is of doubtful value. Clonidine is little better than a placebo. Verapamil and nifedipine may be effective.

Cluster headache (migraineous neuralgia)
1. Ergotamine tartrate 1–2 mg may terminate an attack but attacks usually too short lived for acute treatment. This is the only indication for prophylactic ergotamine tartrate (1–2 mg daily for 1–2 weeks only).
2. Prophylactic lithium carbonate (perhaps a lower plasma level than depression: 0.6–0.7 mmol/l may be effective).
3. A single oral dose of prednisolone (30 mg) may prevent a cluster of headaches from continuing.

DRUGS IN ALZHEIMER'S DISEASE

The disease is probably a result of selective degeneration of cholinergic pathways. The drug strategies include:

Precursor loading: e.g. lecithin — but ineffective.

Stimulation of acetylcholine release: 4-aminopyridine is possibly helpful but causes agitation. Piracetam, oxiracetam and pramiracetam also cause stimulation.

Anticholinesterases: phyostigmine may give a small and brief improvement in cognition. Tetrahydroaminoacridine has no proven benefit.

Cholinergic agonists: arecoline, RS 86, bethanechol all may have some benefit.

Other drugs: selegiline may improve mood and cognitive performance. Co-dergocrine mesylate produces some benefit in apathetic patients.

MYASTHENIA GRAVIS

Associated with serum IgG antibody binding to acetylcholine receptors in muscle, with loss of receptors.

Diagnosis
1. Edrophonium chloride (Tensilon) test: Inject 1–2 mg i.v. of this short-acting anticholinesterase. If no side effects occur then 5–8 mg is given. Positive test is clinical improvement: wears off after 5 mins.
2. Detection of anti-AChR antibody and anti-striated muscle antibody.

Treatment
1. Anticholinesterases: allow acetylcholine released by nerve to act for longer.
   a. *Pyridostigmine* 60 mg 6–8 hourly increasing to 120 mg 3-hourly. Mild GI effect. Contains quaternary nitrogen and is charged at all pH so poorly and slowly absorbed: may be usefully combined with faster absorbed neostigmine for patients weak on waking. *Distigmine* has a more prolonged action, but may cumulate and cause a cholinergic crisis.
   b. *Neostigmine* 15 mg 6–8-hourly but often more frequently (300 mg/day; up to 2-hourly intervals). Short (2–6 h) duration of action. Pronounced muscarinic activity so needs atropine or propantheline to prevent colic and salivation.
2. Steroids indicated if (a) poor response to anticholinergic drugs and/or thymectomy; (b) in older males.

Begin with low dose (or weakness worsens), e.g. prednisolone 10 mg; increase by 5–10 mg/week until symptoms controlled or 120 mg maximum reached. Anticholinergics usually reduced during steroid therapy. Steroids can be combined with azathioprine for most severe disease.
3. Other immunosuppresants: azathioprine.
4. Thymectomy.
5. Plasmapheresis — removes antibody.

Myasthenic crisis: deterioration in myasthenia can be due to infection, or spontaneous. Responds to anticholinesterases.

Cholinergic crisis: deterioration caused by excess anticholinesterase treatment. Worsened by edrophonium. Treated by withdrawal of anticholinesterase. Atropine used to block excessive muscarinic effect.

Drugs which interfere with neuromuscular transmission (myasthenics therefore more sensitive)
1. Aminoglycosides
2. Other antibiotics — Viomycin
                     — Colistin
                     — Polymyxin
3. Antiarrhythmics — Quinidine
                     — Lignocaine
4. Muscle relaxants — Curare
   (but less sensitive to succinylcholine)
5. Respiratory depressants, e.g. barbiturates.

9. Analgesics — including terminal care

OPIOIDS (OPIATES; NARCOTIC ANALGESICS)

These act by binding to opiate receptors in CNS.
Opiate receptors found in:
pulvinar of thalamus
limbic system and connections
midbrain periaqueductal grey matter (gives rise to descending
antinociceptive pathways)
substantia gelatinosa of cord.
Receptor agonists are stereospecific (l-isomers are active) and
competively antagonised by naloxone.
Endogenous analgesic peptides also bind to these receptors:
Met-encephalin and β endorphin (found in periaqueductal grey matter),
met-encephalin also in substantia gelatinosa and raphé nucleus.
The receptors are of several types:
μ : mediate euphoria, dependence, supraspinal analgesia, gut stasis,
meiosis, profound respiratory depression
K : dysphoria, hallucinations, meiosis, less severe respiratory
depression

Actions of morphine (effects lasts 3–4 hours)
A. CNS
Relief of pain — esp. prolonged. Raises pain threshold and
reduces emotional reaction to pain
Euphoria — not seen in normal individuals, but occurs on relief
of pain or removal of withdrawal state
Drowsiness, sleep, coma
Respiratory depression, cough suppression
Vomiting
Convulsions
Pupillary constriction (direct action on Edinger–Westphal nucleus)
Increases release of ADH
Inhibits release of ACTH, FSH, LH
B. Peripheral
Histamine release. Bronchoconstriction in asthmatics
Hypotension

Increased smooth muscle tone
Constipation
Peripheral administration of opioids (e.g. into a joint) may also be analgesic by blocking initiation of ascending nociceptive impulses and reducing peripheral release of substance P.

DRUGS IN TERMINAL CARE

During terminal illness 60% of patients experience pain. Most terminal pain is potentially relieved by drugs. Major analgesic drugs must be given at such intervals (usually 4-hourly) that the effect of the previous dose has not worn off. *Never* prescribe the drugs PRN. Pain itself is hyperalgesic (if necessary the patient must be woken up to be given an analgesic). Analgesics should be given orally whenever possible. Dose increased until patient pain free and memory and fear of pain erased. Constant pain of this type tends to get progressively worse, isolates the patient, demands his whole attention and produces anxiety, depression and fear which themselves potentiate the pain. Treating the isolation, pain, anxiety and depression can break this vicious circle.
Give laxatives with opioids.

PAIN CONTROL

Weaker analgesics
NSAID may be effective in bone pain.
1. *Soluble aspirin* 2–3 × 300 mg tablets 4-hourly.
2. *Paracetamol* 2 × 500 mg tablets 4-hourly.
3. *Co-proxamol* (dextropropoxyphene 32.5 mg plus paracetamol 325 mg) 2 tablets 4-hourly.
   If pain relief does not last up to 4 h, then try nefopam or weak opioids (codeine, dihydrocodeine).

Strong opioids
1. Morphine or diamorphine orally 4-hourly. Increase dose until pain relief attained, then transfer to controlled-release morphine tablets. Alternative strong opioids are buprenorphine, phenazocine and dextromoramide.
2. Neuroleptics given with the narcotic analgesic to potentiate anguish-relieving properties of latter and as antiemetics.
3. Oxycodone pectinate suppositories if vomiting.
4. If injections are needed, diamorphine can be given intermittently or continuously subcutaneously.

Vomiting
Haloperidol, metoclopramide, domperidone, cyclizine or methotrimeprazine. Constipation may cause vomiting and should be treated (e.g. by laculose or docusate).

Table 10(a) Opioid analgesics I

Approved name	Analgesic efficacy and dose	Dependance liability	Special features
Pethidine	1/7 potency of morphine but equianalgesic doses produce same degree of respiratory depression and smooth muscle spasm	Said to produce less euphoria than morphine but still powerfully addicting	Absorbed well from gut but 50% first pass metabolism. Can produce vomiting but no constriction of pupil and less cough suppression than morphine
Diamorphine (diacetylmorphine; heroin)	1.5–2.5 × potency of morphine. Oral dose from 2.5–40 mg, s.c. 4–20 mg, i.v. 1–5 mg	Said to produce more euphoria than morphine hence bigger dependance risk	More active than morphine because enters brain more rapidly. In CNS converted to monoacetylmorphine and morphine. Action lasts ~ 3 hours (but $T_{1/2}$ = 3 mins). Possibly less vomiting than morphine. Enters fetus more readily than morphine
Dextromoramide	Equivalent to morphine 5–20 mg oral or injection	Similar to morphine	Duration of action 3–4 hours. Less sedating than morphine.
Codeine (methylmorphine)	One tenth activity of morphine — but high doses cannot be tolerated. 15–50 mg oral, up to 4-hourly. Injection: 15–60 mg	Uncommon	Used for mild pain, cough suppression and symptomatic control of diarrhoea. Releases low levels of morphine into plasma and brain ($T_{1/2}$ = 2½ h). Injection may be useful in moderate pain

Table 10(b) Opioid analgesics II

Approved name	Analgesic efficacy and dose	Dependance liability	Special features
Dihydrocodeine	Similar to or more potent than codeine	Uncommon	Mild to moderate pain and cough suppression
Diphenoxylate	2.5 mg/tablet Lomotil 4 tablets initially, then 2, 6-hourly	Can occur with prolonged use. May produce euphoria	Use limited to symptomatic treatment of acute self-limiting diarrhoea
Methadone	Similar to morphine oral or injection 5–15 mg (45 min delay in onset after oral)	Less euphoria than morphine. Less severe withdrawal syndrome	Similar analgesic to morphine and used to replace morphine and diamorphine in addicts. Prolonged action
Dipipanone In diconal (10 mg dipipanone + 30 mg cyclizine)	2½ × activity of morphine. 10–25 mg i.m. injection. Diconal given orally	Similar to morphine	Powerful orally active analgesic. Cyclizine causes sedation

Anorexia
Prednisolone (enteric coated) 5–15 mg daily.

Malignant large bowel obstruction
Analgesics plus docusate sodium (Dioctyl forte 1–2 tablets 8 hourly) until obstruction is complete. Lomotil 2 tablets 6-hourly.

Dyspnoea
1. Bronchodilators: salbutamol tablets
                     aminophylline suppositories.
2. Steroids: start at 45 mg prednisolone daily and reduce to 15 mg daily.
3. Antibacterials: cotrimoxazole or ampicillin if dyspnoea accompanied by cough or other evidence of infection
4. If large effusions or neoplastic invasion of lung narcotic analgesics must be used to relieve distress.
5. If excessive secretions and noisy breathing, hyoscine dries secretions and quietens breathing.

Depression and anxiety
1. Prednisolone 5–15 mg daily may greatly improve mood.

Table 10(c) Opioid analgesics III

Approved Name	Analgesic efficacy and dose	Dependence liability	Special features
Oxycodone	30 mg suppository at night (equivalent to 20 mg morphine orally)	Similar to morphine	Useful for night-long analgesia
Phenazocine	3–4 × activity of morphine. 5 mg orally or sublingually 4–6 hourly	Similar to morphine	Similar analgesics to morphine
Pentazocine	½ activity of morphine 25–100 mg oral 3–4 hourly. 30–60 mg i.m., s.c. or i.v. injection	Less dependence than morphine	Partial opiate agonist. Usefulness limited by frequent dysphoric reactions. Not for myocardial infarction
Buprenorphine	15 × activity of morphine. 0.3–0.6 i.m. or slow i.v. injection 6–8-hourly. Sublingual tablet	Less dependence than morphine	Partial opiate agonist. Powerful analgesic not readily reversed by naloxone
Nalbuphine	Injection 10–20 mg	Less dependence than morphine	Partial agonist. Less nausea than morphine. Effect lasts 4–5 hours. Fewer psychotomimetic effects than pentazocine
Meptazinol	Oral and injection tablets 200 mg injection 100 mg	Less dependence than pentazocine	Partial agonist. Causes nausea. Fewer psychotomimetic effects than pentazocine

2. Relief of physical distress.
3. Tricyclic antidepressants, e.g. amitriptyline 25–100 mg daily.
4. If anxiety is dominant: dothiepin 75–100 mg at night. i.v. diazepam 5–20 mg for panic states.

Skeletal metastases
Add aspirin, naproxen or indomethacin to narcotic analgesic treatment. Other measures may be required (e.g. radiotherapy, phenol

nerve block). Salmon calcitonin, four doses given over 2 days may produce prolonged relief.

Cough
1. Linctus methadone 5–10 ml (2 mg/5 ml) at night
2. Antibacterials
3. Bromhexine 8 mg tds to liquify tenacious sputum
4. Diamorphine if the above are not effective.

Itch
1. Chlorpheniramine 4 mg 8-hourly
2. Local or systemic steroids
3. Cholestyramine if biliary obstruction.

Hiccough
1. Metoclopramide 10 mg oral or i.m.
2. Chlorpromazine 25 mg oral or i.m.

NON-STEROIDAL ANTI-INFLAMMATORY DRUGS (NSAID)

Act peripherally and centrally on cyclooxygenase and block prostaglandin synthesis. Aspirin causes irreversible acetylation of serine residues in platelet cyclooxygenase.

Shared properties of NSAID
1. Anti-inflammatory, antipyretic, analgesic.
2. Inhibition of platelet aggregation.
3. Gastric irritation, ulceration and haemorrhage. Aggravate peptic ulcer. Antagonised by misoprostol and H_2 antagonists
4. Hypersensitivity reactions are common.
5. Elevation of plasma creatinine and urea and shedding of epithelial cells in urine after brief drug exposure. Can cause acute reduction in GFR, acute interstitial nephritis or acute renal failure. Long term use can produce structural damage and chronic renal failure (analgesic nephropathy).
6. (Probable) hepatic damage.
7. Prolongation of labour.
8. Potentiation of effects of anticoagulants (esp. azapropazone and aspirin. Naproxen and ibuprofen do not prolong prothrombin time).
9. Sodium and water retention, hyponatraemia, hyperkalaemia.

ASPIRIN

Pharmacokinetics
1. Low doses: First order elimination, 80% converted to salicylurate.
2. High doses saturate this conjugation reaction and thus eliminated by zero order kinetics, so $T_{1/2}$ changes with dose.

3. V_d reduced in patients with R.A.
4. 80–85% bound to plasma protein.

Toxicity
1. Asymptomatic blood loss, haematemesis and malaena, nausea, vomiting, exacerbation of peptic ulceration.
2. Hypersensitivity:
   a. asthmatic attacks in patients with nasal polyps
   b. urticaria and angioedema.
3. Salicylism: tinnitus, deafness, nausea, vomiting and abdominal pain.
4. Gout (urate retention with low doses, urate elimination with high doses).
5. Transient decrease in renal function.
6. Aggravation of bleeding disorders.
7. Hepatotoxicity uncommon; abnormal LFT common.
8. Delayed onset of labour. ?Small for dates babies associated with aspirin use in pregnancy.
9. Reye's syndrome: encephalopathy and fatty change in organs (esp. liver) in young children with a febrile illness given aspirin. Rare. 50% die.
10. Drug interactions:
    potentiation of gastric irritants
    potentiation of hypoglycaemics
    potentiation of anticoagulants

Table 11 NSAID: aspirin group

Drug	Tolerability	Special uses
Aspirin Soluble aspirin	Excellent in acute illness. Gastric irritation with full doses on prolonged use	Long term prophylaxis of occlusive vascular disease (dose 30 mg/day)
Aloxiprin (buffered aspirin) Enteric-coated aspirin Slow release aspirin Choline magnesium trisalicylate Benorylate (aspirin-paracetamol ester which dissociates after absorption)	Better tolerated than plain aspirin on prolonged use. Additional paracetamol should not be given with benorylate	
Diflunisal	Better tolerated than aspirin but avoid in peptic ulceration	

reduces effects of steroids
reduces effects of diuretics and antihypertensives.

Uses
1. Non-specific musculo-skeletal pain and soft tissue rheumatism.
2. Febrile illnesses and mild/moderate pain. Severe pain e.g. bony metastases.
3. Rheumatoid arthritis.
4. Acute rheumatism and other acute and subacute arthropathies.
5. Osteoarthritis.
6. Long term prevention of thrombotic disease and probably other occlusive vascular disease. 30 mg aspirin/day carries less risk of brain and GI haemorrhage than 300 mg/d.
7. Control of radiation-induced diarrhoea.
8. I.M. diclofenac effective in biliary and renal colic.

Other drugs for rheumatic diseases

i.m. sodium aurothiomalate p.o. auranofin Penicillamine Chloroquine and hydroxychloroquine Sulphasalazine	slow or reverse progress of rheumatoid arthritis, juvenile rheumatism, palindromic rheumatism and lupus erythematosus
Colchicine Probenecid and sulphinpyrazone Allopurinol	for acute gout uricosurics for chronic gout xanthine oxidase inhibitor for chronic gout

RHEUMATOID ARTHRITIS (RA)

Physiotherapy, splinting, NSAID, other analgesics (and steroids) relieve pain, reduce swelling and stiffness in RA but do not influence the progress of joint destruction and other tissue damage.

Disease-modifying drugs include gold, penicillamine, sulphasalazine, hydroxychloroquine and immunosuppressants. These reduce pain, improve mobility, reduce ESR and C-reactive protein, reduce vasculitis and possibly slow down erosive joint damage. Most patients respond to low dose methotrexate. Sulphasalazine is also effective in seronegative arthritis including ankylosing spondylitis.

Sodium aurothiomalate
Toxicity includes: mouth ulcers, rash, nephrotic syndrome, blood disorders, colitis.

Auranofin
Causes diarrhoea more commonly, but other toxic effects less
frequently than aurothiomalate.

Penicillamine
Can cause mouth ulcers, loss of taste, hypersensitivity rash,
agranulocytosis and thrombocytopenia

Table 12 NSAID: some alternative agents

Approved name	Pharmacokinetics	Tolerability	Clinical features
Phenylacetic acid derivatives			
Diclofenac	Can depress plasma salicylate levels. $T\frac{1}{2} = 1$–2 h	Rashes and GI disturbances	Intramuscular administration for renal colic. Similar to naproxen
Phenylpropionic acid derivatives			
Ibuprofen	$T\frac{1}{2} = 2$ h	Low incidence of side effects	Weak anti-inflammatory actions
Ketoprofen	Slow release form available. $T\frac{1}{2} = 2\frac{1}{2}$ h	More toxic than ibuprofen	As effective as ibuprofen
Naproxen	Non-linear protein binding in high doses. $T\frac{1}{2} = 12$–15 h	Low incidence of side effects	Useful in acute gout. A powerful NSAID of first choice
Flurbiprofen			
Fenbufen	Prodrug: at least 2 active metabolites with long half-lives are produced in the liver. No accumulation in moderate renal failure. $T\frac{1}{2} = 3$–6 h	High risk of rashes	Single daily dose. Similar efficacy to naproxen
Oxicam			
Piroxicam	No evidence of altered metabolism in elderly. $T\frac{1}{2} = 36$–100 h.	Well tolerated	Single daily dose. Can be used in acute gout

Chloroquine and hydroxychloroquine
Are better tolerated than gold and penicillamine but can cause ocular toxicity. Retinopathy is rare if the standard doses are not exceeded and if the drugs are not given continuously for longer than 2 years.

NON OPIOID, NON ANTI-INFLAMMATORY ANALGESICS

Paracetamol
Has similar analgesic efficacy to aspirin, even in rheumatic disease. Safer than NSAID on gastric mucosa. Overdose causes vomiting in

Table 13 NSAID: pyrazolone group

Drug	Pharmacokinetics	Toxicity	Clinical features
Phenylbutazone	Completely absorbed orally. Small V_d; 98% protein bound. 99% metabolised to oxyphenbutazone and to the C-glucuronide. $T_{1/2}$ = 2–4 days	Rashes and GI disturbances common. Agranulocytosis rare. Salt and water retention. Jaundice. Drug interactions	Highly effective anti-inflammatory agents, but reserved for acute gout and intractable ankylosing spondylitis because of toxicity
Oxyphenbutazone	$T_{1/2}$ = 1–2 days		Oxyphenbutazone eye ointment used in episcleritis, scleritis and anterior uveitis
Azapropazone	Well absorbed orally. Not extensively metabolised. $T_{1/2}$ = 1 day. 98% protein bound	Rashes and GI disturbances	Effective analgesics and anti-inflammatory agents. Azaprazone used in acute gout

Table 14 NSAID: anthranilic acid derivatives

Approved name	Pharmacokinetics	Toxicity	Clinical features
Mefenamic acid	Slow absorption from gut (peak at 2–3 h) 99% bound to plasma proteins	Diarrhoea is common. Less common: dizziness, rashes, leucopenia, autoimmune haemolysis	Analgesic, weak anti-inflammatory

Table 15 NSAID: Indoleacetic acid derivatives

Approved name	Pharmacokinetics	Toxicity	Clinical features
Sulindac	Given as sulphoxide (inactive) is rapidly absorbed. Metabolised to sulphide (active). $T\frac{1}{2} = 16$ h. Enterohepatic circulation	Less gastric irritation, less CNS toxicity than indomethacin. Constipation common	Similar profile to naproxen
Tolmetin	Well and rapidly absorbed. Highly protein bound. $T\frac{1}{2} = 1$ h. Excreted in urine partly unchanged, partly metabolised and conjugated. Metabolism accelerated when given with aspirin	GI disturbances common. Headache and dizziness	Similar profile to ibuprofen
Indomethacin	Rapidly absorbed from small intestine and rectum. $T\frac{1}{2} = 7$ h, but more prolonged action	Headaches giddiness and GI toxicity	Effective as naproxen but more toxic. Also used to close a persistent ductus

first 2 days and potentially hepatic and renal failure after 3–5 days. Poisoning is severe if blood level is above 70 mg/l at 10 h. Treated with oral methionine or i.v. N-acetylcysteine as early as possible.

Nefopam
Is sometimes effective in persistent pain which has not responded to NSAID. It causes negligible respiratory depression but has anticholinergic and sympathomimetic side effects.

10. Drugs for cardiovascular disease

ANGINA PECTORIS

Angina pectoris: referred pain from an ischaemic myocardium. Much (but not all) angina is due to atherosclerotic coronary artery disease.

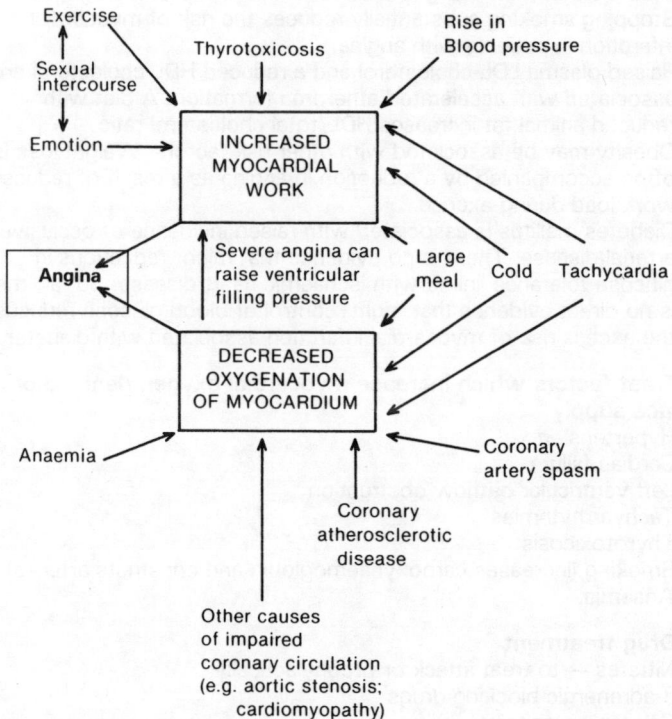

Fig. 10.1 Scheme of factors producing angina.

MANAGEMENT OF ANGINA

Patients with recent onset of angina merit investigation with exercise test and angiography in order to decide about surgical treatment (bypass/angioplasty).

A. Risk factors which can be manipulated
1. Insufficient exercise
2. Hypertension
3. Smoking
4. Plasma lipids
5. Obesity
6. Abnorml glucose tolerance.

1. Physical activity must not be curtailed. A graded exercise program should be recommended in medically managed patients and after successful surgery.
2. Hypertension must be controlled.
3. Stop smoking. Smoking is prothrombotic and proatherogenic. Stopping smoking substantially reduces the risk of myocardial infarction in patients with angina.
4. Raised plasma LDL-cholesterol and a reduced HDL-cholesterol are associated with accelerated atheroma formation. A diet with reduced animal fat increases HDL/total cholesterol ratio.
5. Obesity may be associated with other risk factors. Weight loss is often accompanied by a reduction in angina as a result of reduced work load during exerice.
6. Diabetes mellitus is associated with raised incidence of occlusive arterial disease. There is no evidence that minor reductions in glucose tolerance linked with ischaemic heart disease. So far, there is no direct evidence that 'tight' control of blood glucose reduces the excess risk of myocardial infarction associated with diabetes.

B. Treat factors which increase myocardial oxygen demand or reduce supply
1. Hypertension
2. Cardiac failure
3. Left ventricular outflow obstruction
4. Tachyarrhythmias
5. Thyrotoxicosis
6. Smoking (increases carboxyhaemoglobin and constricts arteries)
7. Anaemia.

C. Drug treatment
1. Nitrates — to treat attack or prophylactically
2. β-adrenergic blocking drugs
3. Calcium antagonist
4. Aspirin. Does not influence the symptom of angina, but reduces the risk of myocardial infarction, especially in unstable angina.

NITRATES

a. **Glyceryl trinitrate** — sublingually during attack
                            — prophylactically before exercise.

Vasodilator — mainly veins. It is metabolised to nitric oxide which is also synthesised from endogenous substrates by endothelial cells: 'endothelium–derived relaxing factor'. Nitric oxide activates guanylate cyclase in vascular smooth muscle, forming cGMP which causes relaxation by sequestration of cytoplasmic Ca^{2+}, and increasing K^+ conductance of the cell membrane.
Plasma $T_{1/2} \sim 2$–3 min. Action begins within 2 min and lasts up to 30 min.
Given *sublingually* because:
1. High first-pass hepatic metabolism ($\sim$80–90%) to inactive metabolites when given orally.
2. Rapid buccal absorption.
Tell patient:
 (i) about possible side effects (see below)
 (ii) not to put tablets in sunlight, in bottles with other tablets or cotton wool (glyceryl trinitrate is volatile and absorbs on to other materials from tablet). Keep the cap screwed on tight, and the bottle away from direct heat.
(iii) to check expiry date of tablets
(iv) use prophylactically
 (v) effect terminated by swallowing or spitting out tablet.

Other routes of administration
Transdermal glyceryl trinitrate (Transiderm-Nitro) — self-adhesive plastic patch which is applied to the skin (usually applied to the lateral chest) once every 24 h.
Spray — measured dose onto tongue.

Sustained-action glyceryl trinitrate tablets
Evidence of beneficial effect used at maximum dosage.

Adverse effects
Headache
Palpitations and tachycardia — may paradoxically exacerbate angina
Postural hypotension
Chronic high doses rarely cause methaemoglobinaemia
Tolerance is very common. Its mechanism is not understood, but possibly relates to failure to convert organic nitrate to nitric oxide because of depletion of a sulphydryl cofactor. Avoided by omitting the night–time dose when possible.

Contraindications
1. Hypertrophic obstructive cardiomyopathy — nitrates increase outflow tract obstruction.

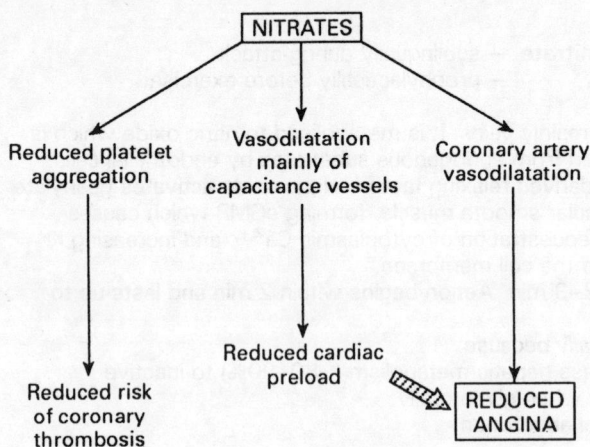

Fig. 10.2 Actions of nitrates in angina pectoris.

2. Cor pulmonale — increase hypoxaemia by venous admixture.

Long acting nitrates
1. Isosorbide dinitrate
    — sublingual — can be used for acute attack
    — chewable
    — slow release (Isoket Retard).
2. Isosorbide 5-mononitrate — major active metabolite produced by first-pass metabolism of isosorbide dinitrate.

β-BLOCKERS

Reduce cardiac oxygen demand by:
1. reducing heart rate
2. reducing blood pressure on exercise
3. depressing contractility.
    Can be used in combination with nitrates.
    Atypical (Prinzmetal) angina rarely responds, and may worsen, with β-blockers (probably due to a unopposed coronary vasoconstrictor α-activity).
NB
1. Sudden withdrawal of β-blockers may increase angina or precipitate myocardial infarction.
2. β-blockers reduce risk of reinfarction after recovery from a transmural infarct.
Contraindications (see p. 120)

CALCIUM ANTAGONISTS

Blockade of voltage-activated slow calcium channels causes:
1. peripheral arteriolar dilation and hence reduced cardiac afterload
2. coronary artery vasodilation
3. reduced activity in pacemaker nodal tissue in the atria
4. decreased speed and force of cardiac contraction.

Particularly useful for:
1. With nitrates when β-blocker contraindicated
2. Atypical (Prinzmetal) angina and coronary spasm.

Diltiazem vasodilates without tachycardia, but nifedipine usually causes reflex tachycardia.

Other Ca^{2+} antagonists which are effective in both angina and hypertension: verapamil, isradipine and lamodipine.

Use of combined oral preparations of Ca^{2+} antagonists with β-blockers has not been found to be more effective than the use of either drug class alone (although combinations are manufactured). Both are negatively inotropic and the combination can precipitate heart failure.

SECONDARY PREVENTION IN SURVIVORS OF MYOCARDIAL INFARCTION

1. Stop smoking.
2. Regular physical activity.
3. Control hypertension, obesity, diabetes mellitus.
4. Treat hypercholesterolaemia.
5. Drug treatment:
   a. β-blockers reduce rate of sudden death especially if begun as soon as possible after infarction.
      Propranolol, timolol, metoprolol, oxprenolol all shown to be effective.
   b. Platelet active drugs. Aspirin reduces rate of reinfarction.
   c. Calcium channel blockers. Diltiazem may reduce the risk of reinfarction, especially following subendocardial infarcts, where it could be preferable to β-blockers.

CARDIAC FAILURE

Occurs when heart unable to pump blood at the rate required for systemic metabolic requirements during normal activity. Mortality akin to some malignancies: 5 year survival about 50%.

$$\text{Cardiac output} = \text{Heart rate} \times \text{Stroke volume}$$

Stroke Volume determined by:
1. *Filling pressure* ('Pre-load'). Frank-Starling ventricular function curve shows that stroke volume increases with increasing LV filling pressure.

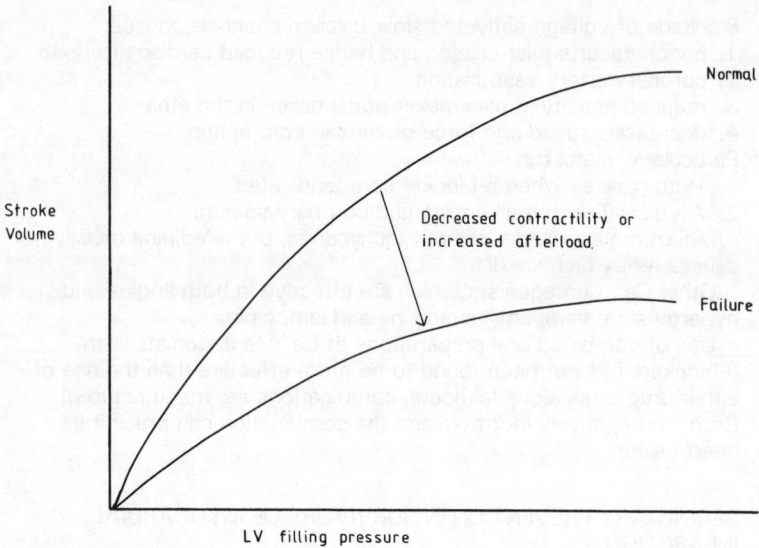

Fig. 10.3

2. *Afterload* depends on intraventricular pressure and ventricular volume and is equivalent to tension in ventricular wall during contraction. Ventricular volume determined by aortic impedance (roughly equivalent to peripheral resistance). Myocardial disease depresses the ventricular function curve.

3. *Contractility (inotropic state) of myocardium* — decrease depresses ventricular function curves (see Fig. 10.4)

In failure the underlying condition usually decreases contractility. Consequent increases in heart rate, preload and afterload (via activation of sympathetic autonomic and renin-angiotensin-aldosterone systems). May be counter-regulatory (i.e. make the situation worse, not better).

Principles of management of cardiac failure

Heart rate can rarely be beneficially manipulated. Recent attempts to exploit the effects of a partial β-agonist (xamoterol) on heart rate and contractility illustrate the problems: patients with mild heart failure experienced some benefit, whereas those with more severe disease were made worse. Since the natural history of cardiac failure is progressive deterioration, the potential usefulness of such a drug is limited.

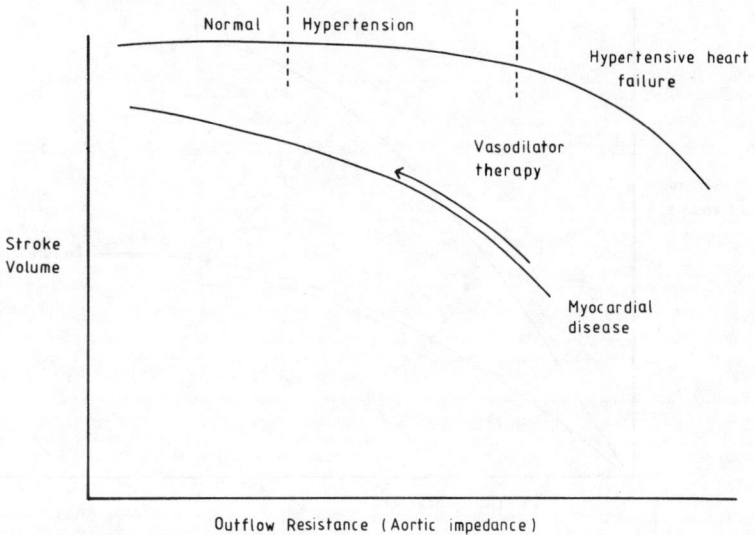

Outflow Resistance (Aortic impedance)

Fig. 10.4

1. Correction of underlying disease, e.g. thyrotoxicosis, valvular dysfunction.
2. Reduction of cardiac workload: control hypertension (diuretics, converting enzyme inhibitors) and obesity.
3. Reduce sodium intake and avoid drugs producing fluid retention, e.g. indomethacin.
4. Diuretics: reduce overexpanded extracellular fluid volume: reduce filling pressure without increased output (F → B) but stroke volume may later rise due to slowly improving ventricular function (→ C). In acute failure early response to loop diuretics due to vasodilation.
5. Inotropic agents increase contractility, e.g. digitalis, dopamine, dobutamine and shift curves up and to left (→ D).

    Oral phosphodiesterase inhibitors (e.g. milrinone) are being investigated as inotropes, but their place (if any) remains to be established.
6. Vasodilators. *Venous dilators* (e.g. isosorbide mononitrate) reduce filling pressure (F → V).

    Decrease (LV) volume, ventricular diameter and so wall tension and thus oxygen demand (large hearts consume more oxygen).

    Arterial dilators (e.g. prazosin)

    Reduce impedance so cardiac output increases and shift Frank-Starling curve (F → A).

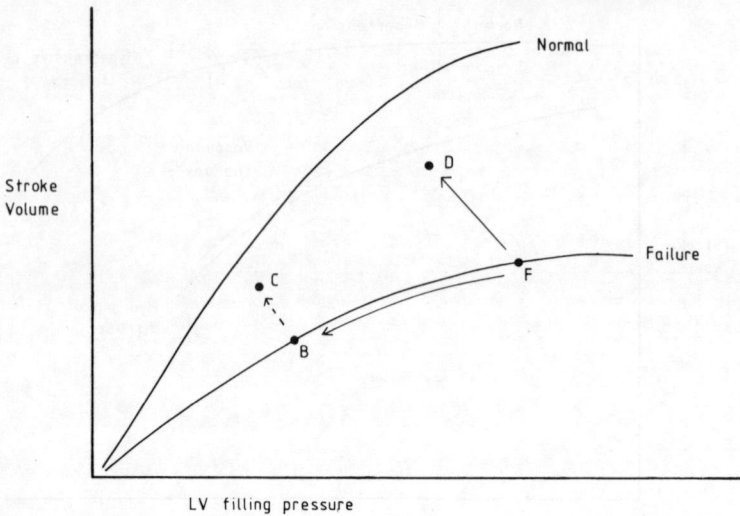

Fig. 10.5

Reduce myocardial oxygen consumption because reduce LV wall tension.

Combined pre- and afterload reduction
This is achieved by angiotensin converting enzyme inhibitors (ACE-I) such as captopril and enalapril. These are now the drugs of choice in this category, and have been shown to prolong life in patients with chronic heart failure. Diuretics are withheld for a day to reduce the risk of first-dose hypotension. For the same reason the first dose of ACE-I is small and is given at night. Potassium retention (due to reduced aldosterone) is usually mild, but may be a problem if potassium-retaining diuretics are used (e.g. amiloride in 'Moduretic' and 'Frumil') especially if there is renal impairment. Plasma potassium and creatinine should be monitored.

Acute failure
Sit up; give oxygen
Loop diuretic
Morphine or diamorphine
Nitrates may be effective
   Monitoring pressures in the right chambers of the heart (Swan–Ganz technique) may be indicated and guide therapy such as volume replacement and use of positive inotropes (such as dobutamine).

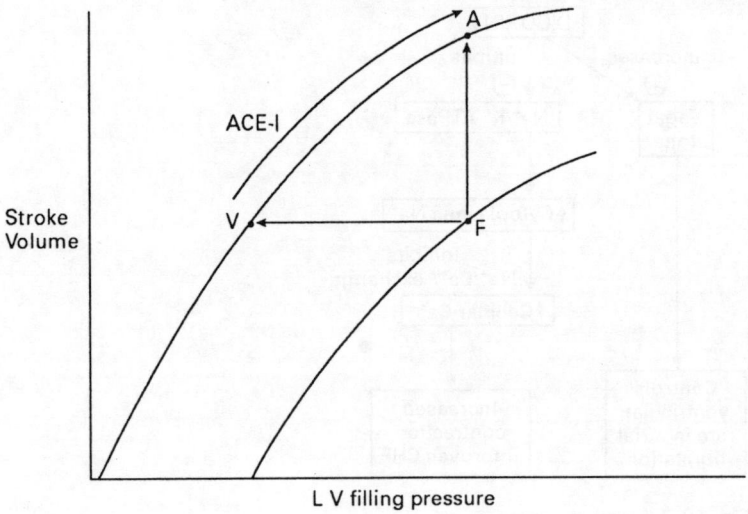

Fig. 10.6

Chronic failure
Treat cause
Reduce alcohol and salt intake
Diuretic (e.g. frusemide)
ACE inhibitors
? digoxin.

DIGITALIS GLYCOSIDES

Digoxin most commonly used.

Uses
1. Fast atrial fibrillation
2. Atrial flutter
3. Supraventricular tachycardia
4. Congestive heart failure — but benefit is small in patients in sinus
   rhythm.

PHARMACOKINETICS OF DIGOXIN

Absorption from gut   Variable
                      20–80%
                      (bioavailability may be a therapeutic problem)

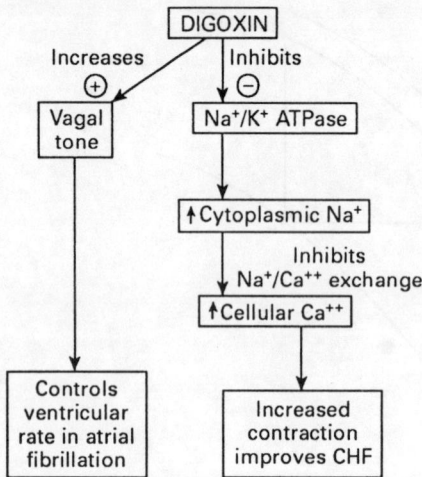

Fig. 10.7 Mode of action.

Hepatic metabolism	Minimal
Renal excretion	80% (a relatively polar drug)
Protein binding	25%
Lipid solubility	Relatively low (therefore obese patients should not be dosed on the basis of their body weight)
T½	approximately 1 day
Approx. therapeutic levels (nmol/l)	1–2.5
Source	*Digitalis lanata* (white foxglove)

TOXICITY OF CARDIAC GLYCOSIDES

Narrow therapeutic range: toxicity seen in 15–20% unselected patients and is potentially fatal.

A. Gastrointestinal
Common — anorexia, nausea, vomiting — probably via central effect on chemoreceptor trigger zone in medulla.
Uncommon — diarrhoea, constipation, abdominal pain.
Rare — haemorrhagic bowel necrosis.

B. Cardiovascular
May not be preceded by GI effects.
First degree heart block is sometimes premonitory of more serious

arrhythmias. Commonest effects are sinus bradycardia; nodal rhythm, bigeminal rhythm (paired ventricular extrasystoles), but any type of arrhythmia or conduction defect may occur.
Less commonly — cardiac arrest.

C. neurological
Common — headache, drowsiness, fatigue, acute confusional state, blurred vision, altered colour vision, visual aberrations.
Rare — neuralgia, paraesthesiae, coma, optic neuritis producing scotomata or blindness, paresis of ocular muscles, muscular weakness.

D. Others
Rare — rashes due to allergy, gynaecomastia.

PREDISPOSING FACTORS TO DIGOXIN INTOXICATION

1. Electrolyte disturbance
Hypokalaemia
Hypercalcaemia.

2. Disease states
Renal failure — impaired excretion
Hypothyroidism — prolonged $T_{1/2}$, reduced V_d
Hypoxia — sensitises to arrhythmias.

3. Old age
Reduced renal function also decreased muscle mass relative to body fat reduces volume of distribution.

Failure of treatment in heart failure
1. Poor compliance.
2. Excessive salt intake.
3. Inadequate dosage.
4. Concurrent use of drugs producing heart failure (see below).
5. Severe splanchnic venous congestion reducing bioavailability of oral diuretics — try parenteral administration.
6. Secondary hyperaldosteronism.
7. Water retention with hyponatraemia — usually a sign of severe underlying disease.

Drug-induced heart failure
1. Myocardial depression
   a. Reversible
      (i) β-adrenergic blockers
      (ii) disopyramide — other anti-arrhythmics (lignocaine, mexilitine, quinidine, procainamide) only rarely cause failure in usual dosage

(iii) Calcium ion antagonists (nifedipine, verapamil) occasionally cause failure, especially if β-blockers used
   b. Irreversible
      (i) cytotoxic agents — anthracyclines (related to cumulative dose); cyclophosphamide (high doses)
      (ii) alcohol (cardiomyopathy)
      (iii) emetine
      (iv) chloroquine.
2. Salt and water retention (also aggravate hypertension)
   a. Non-steroidal anti-inflammatory drugs
   b. Corticosteroids and ACTH
   c. Oestrogens
   d. Carbenoxolone
   e. Chlorpropamide
   f. Sodium containing drugs — some antacids, carbenicillin sodium, some X-ray contrast media (e.g. Conray 420).

CARDIAC ARRHYTHMIAS

Life threatening cardiac arrhythmias are often treated non-pharmacologically (e.g. electrical defibrillation, DC shock for ventricular fibrillation, ventricular tachycardia or supraventricular tachyarrhythmias associated with cardiovascular collapse, cardiac pacing for complete heart block).

Vaughan Williams classification
Based on micro-electrode studies. Most agents increase effective refractory period, thereby preventing re-entry depolarisation.

Class I ('membrane stabilising action' — a local anaesthetic property)
Reduce rate of rise (dV/dt) of phase 0 by inhibiting Na^+ entry through fast channel.
   a. increase duration of action potential.
      — quinidine
      — procainamide
      — disopyramide
   b. decrease duration of action potential
      — lignocaine
      — mexiletine
      — phenytoin
      — tocainide
   c. no effect on duration of action potential
      — lorcainide

Class II
β-blockers such as atenolol, metoprolol and sotalol.

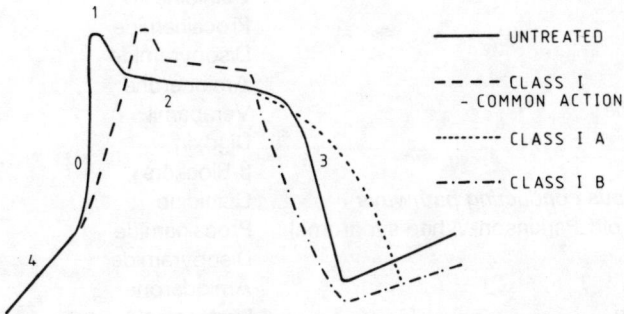

Fig. 10.8

Class III
Prolong duration of action potential without much effect on dV/dt of phase 0, e.g. amiodarone, D-sotalol.

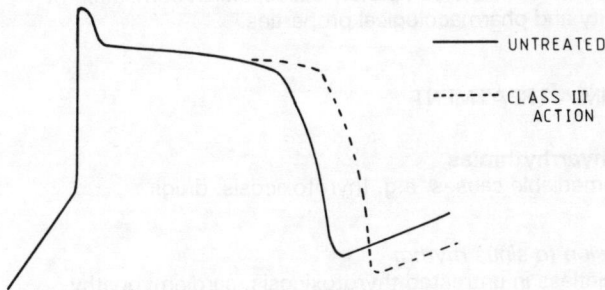

Fig. 10.9

Class IV
Verapamil and diltiazem block slow inward Ca^{++} current. A-V node (where this current produces major depolarisation) particularly sensitive. NB A-V node is part of re-entry circuit for many paroxysmal supraventricular tachycardias.

Clinical classification
Effects on type of cardiac tissue supporting arrhythmia.

Sinus node   β-blockers
                                Verapamil
                                Digoxin

Atrium	Quinidine
	Procainamide
	Disopyramide
	Amiodarone
A-V node	Verapamil
	Digoxin
	β-Blockers
Anomalous conducting pathways	Quinidine
(as in Wolff-Parkinson-White syndrome)	Procainamide
	Disopyramide
	Amiodarone
Ventricle	Lignocaine
	Mexiletine
	Phenytoin
	Quinidine
	Procainamide
	Disopyramide
	Amiodarone

Note: No classification is completely successful in correlation of clinical utility and pharmacological properties.

ARRHYTHMIA TREATMENT

Atrial tachyarrhythmias
Exclude remediable causes, e.g. thyrotoxicosis, drugs.

1. Conversion to sinus rhythm
Usually pointless in untreated thyrotoxicosis, cardiomyopathy, rheumatic heart disease because early recurrence likely.
   Vagal stimulation, e.g. carotid sinus massage, Valsalva manoeuvre, may terminate paroxysmal atrial tachycardia.
   If circulation compromised by arrhythmia (systolic BP < 80 mmHg; cold extremities; clouded consciousness; sweating; oliguria; pulmonary oedema) proceed to DC cardioversion immediately. Synchronised DC shocks (50–400 J) necessary (unsynchronised shock may produce ventricular fibrillation); start with small charge 25–30 J and increase by 100 J until several 400 J shocks given. Best performed under short-acting i.v. anaesthetic or diazepam 5–20 mg i.v. Relative contraindications: previous digoxin therapy; hypo and hyper-kalaemia.

Cardioversion usually works for atrial tachycardia and flutter but fibrillation may be very resistant. Cardioversion more frequently succeeds if the arrhythmia is of short duration and the atrium is not enlarged. *Elective* cardioversion is preceded by anticoagulation for several weeks to reduce the risk of emboli. It is more likely to be successful if cardiac failure, hypoxaema, metabolic acidosis and potassium imbalances are corrected. Avoid digoxin before attempting cardioversion. Resistant SVT is a serious problem: all drugs except glycosides and amiodarone are negative inotropes and may exacerbate the situation if they fail to control the rate. Transvenous atrial pacing with overpacing of the arrhythmia, may be considered. In broad complex tachycardia of uncertain cause, intravenous adenosine is diagnostically and therapeutically useful.

If control not urgent consider anti-arrhythmic drugs: V-W Class IA and III. First choice is i.v. verapamil.

2. Control of ventricular rate
Symptomatic improvement occurs when ventricular rate controlled.
  If possible, determine AV conduction pathway.
a. Commonly AV node to His-Purkinje system with normal QRS or aberrant conduction. AV node refractoriness increased with verapamil, β-blockers or digoxin so reducing number of impulses transmitted to ventricles. Digoxin still drug of choice for atrial fibrillation (has added effect on conduction down bundle of His). Can add verapamil or β-blocker to initial digoxin therapy if control inadequate. However verapamil raises digoxin levels and thus low doses are used to avoid toxicity. Verapamil and β-blockers should not be mixed.
b. Anomalous conduction pathway present (Wolff-Parkinson-White syndrome). Refractoriness of anomalous pathway unaffected by verapamil or β-blockers. Digoxin may dangerously accelerate conduction in pathway and precipitate tachycardia. It should be avoided in Wolff-Parkinson-White syndrome. Drugs of choice impair atrial and anomalous pathway conduction, e.g. amiodarone.

Some patients are best treated by pathway ablation.

Table 16 Antiarrhythmic drugs

Drug	Dosage	Pharmacokinetics	Adverse effects	Comments
Lignocaine	Slow i.v. bolus 50–100 mg then 4 mg/min for 30 min, 2 mg/min for 2 hrs then 1 mg/min thereafter	Rapid distribution so effect of bolus lasts only a few mins. $T_{1/2}$ 1.5–2 h in normals but increased several-fold by heart or hepatic failure. High hepatic extraction with metabolism to toxic metabolites. Clearance decreased (with elevation of plasma levels) on prolonged (48 + hours) infusion	Paraesthesiae, giddiness, somnolence confusion, fits, myocardial depression	Reduce infusion (not bolus dose) by half in shock, cirrhosis, β-blockade, heart failure (because liver blood flow is low in these cases so lignocaine clearance impaired)
Quinidine	Too dangerous i.v.; p.o. as sulphate – 0.2–0.3 g 3-hourly up to 4 g/day. Long acting bisulphate; given ~ 500 mg 12 hourly – 1st dose preceded by loading dose 0.6–0.8 g sulphate to give therapeutic levels in 3 hours	Plasma levels useful to control dosage and toxicity. (Therapeutic 2.5–5 μg/ml). Hepatic metabolism, $T_{1/2}$ 7–9 h, increased by hepatic and cardiac failure; old age but not renal failure	Depresses intracardiac conduction (stop if QRS >140 secs). Paroxysmal ventricular arrhythmias = quinidine syncope. Diarrhoea and GI upset; vertigo; tinnitus; thrombocytopenic purpura; agranulocytosis. Anticholinergic so usually sinus rate ↑	Dangerous drug. d-isomer of quinine so causes cinchonism. Increases plasma digoxin levels (→ toxicity); enhances hypotensive agents and coumarins; exacerbates myasthenia

Table 16 (continued)

Drug	Dosage	Pharmacokinetics	Adverse effects	Comments
Disopyramide	p.o. 300 mg loading dose then 100–150 mg 6-hourly. Max 200 mg 6-hourly. Sustained release 250–375 mg 12-hourly	50% hepatic metabolism; 50% excreted unchanged in urine. Therapeutic plasma level 2–6 µg/ml	Pronounced anticholinergic effects (dry mouth; urinary retention; glaucoma etc). Occasionally ventricular fibrillation (like quinidine). Negative inotrope — may precipitate cardiac failure	Avoid in heart failure; glaucoma; enlarged prostate
Verapamil	5–10 mg i.v. stat slowly or 5–10 mg by slow infusion over 1 h (max 100 mg/24 h). Orally 40–120 mg 8-hourly	Hypotensive effect disappears by 20 mins but effect on A-V node onset at 10–15 mins and lasts up to 6 h. Oral drug takes 2 h to act. Complete absorption but 80–90% first pass metabolism to norverapamil which has some activity. $T_{1/2}$ 3–7 h	Heart block, asystole, bradycardia, negatively inotropic, hypotension. Side effects rare with oral verapamil (nausea, dizziness, flushing)	Increased bioavailability in cirrhosis (shunting across liver allows higher oral absorption). Cannot give i.v. with β-blocker or digitalis toxicity. Avoid in heart failure; A-V block, sick-sinus syndrome, cardiomegaly

Table 16 (continued)

Drug	Dosage	Pharmacokinetics	Adverse effects	Comments
Amiodarone	200 mg p.o. 8-hourly for at least 1 week — when desired effect occurs dose reduced weekly to minimum dose (usually 200 mg daily)	Very long $T_{1/2}$~28 days so takes long time to reach steady state. Blood levels very low because highly concentrated in tissues. Plasma levels of little clinical value although may be related to toxicity. Response begins after 3–7 days treatment and increases over several weeks	Sinus bradycardia common. Corneal microdeposits (only visible with slit lamp) reversible. T wave becomes notched, lengthened and flattened. Photosensitive rashes. Contains iodine and can cause hypo- or hyperthyroidism. Headaches, nightmares and rarely hepatitis, peripheral neuropathy, tremor, pulmonary alveolitis	Not severely negatively inotropic. Important drug interactions — potentiates warfarin; increases digoxin levels; potentiates bradycardia with β-blockers and verapamil. Contraindicated in sinoatrial and A-V block. Increases digoxin levels (and toxicity)

Ventricular tachyarrhythmias in acute myocardial infarction
Either abnormal focus or re-entry circus mechanism responsible. Often cause of sudden death.

Conversion to sinus rhythm
Exclude and treat remediable causes as soon as possible:

Hypokalaemia (oral or i.v. KCl) — keep K$^+$ between 4.5–5 mmol/l. In problem cases measure magnesium as well.
anoxia and/or acidosis.
pain (use opiate; catheterise distended bladder)
anxiety (reassurance; diazepam).
If circulation is compromised (cardiac arrest) a pre-cordial blow may be effective. Urgent DC cardioversion is necessary.
Anaesthesia may not be necessary if consciousness impaired. Initial shock 150–200 J followed by 300 J then 400 J. If this fails 200–400 mg bretylium tosylate or 100 mg (repeated to total 300 mg) lignocaine i.v. may restore sinus rhythm; if not, shock again.
If ventricular tachycardia rate <170/min and systolic BP >100 mm Hg drugs may be tried before DC cardioversion. Most effective are lignocaine and amiodarone. Lignocaine is commonly used first but there is presently no rational way to select a drug.

Bradycardia after myocardial infarction
Due to excessive vagal activity; hypotensive/syncopal response to opiates; A-V block. Aim to keep rate >50/min if there are symptoms of hypoperfusion.
Atropine 0.3 mg i.v. every 5 mins to maximum 2.4 mg/h and titrate to desired effect. Digoxin, β-blockers and verapamil should be withheld.
Pacing required if bradycardia unresponsive to atropine and severe.
NB isoprenaline is now rarely needed in heart block, but it may be useful in patients with complete heart block during transfer to a unit with facilities for pacing. Its disadvantage is that it increases myocardial oxygen consumption and hence may cause extension of infarction. Its use should be supervised by a physician.

TREATMENT OF SHOCK

Reduced perfusion of essential organs produces tissue hypoxia and derangement of function. Three main types of shock which involve dysfunction of the heart, blood volume and blood flow distribution to varying degree:
1. hypovolaemic — loss of whole blood, plasma or electrolytes
2. cardiogenic — cardiac infarction, tamponade or pulmonary embolism

3. septic — complicates many infections including postoperative.
Main principles are:
1. Optimise pre-load: replace lost blood volume; in postoperative and
myocardial infarction optimal blood volume may be 250–500 ml
greater than normal to get maximum effect from Frank-Starling curve.
According to circumstances blood, plasma, crystalloids (usually large
volumes needed to replace blood loss) or plasma substitutes needed.
Substitutes currently available:
  a. gelatin (degraded to MW of 30 000), e.g. Haemacel
  b. albumin — very expensive.
2. Improve myocardial contractility if output still inadequate when
pre-load optimum:
  a. catecholamines with varying properties (see Table 17)
  b. glucagon — indicated if catecholamines ineffective or
     contraindicated by arrhythmia. Useful in patients suffering from
     β-blockade.
3. Reduce afterload:
   direct acting agents, e.g. nitroprusside
4. Correct metabolic disturbances
— oxygen
5. Antibiotics in septic shock.

Treatment of anaphylactic shock
1a. Adrenaline 0.5–1 mg (0.5–1 ml of 1:1000 adrenaline) given
    intramuscularly. NB: not subcutaneously because absorption slow
    in shock. Repeat every 15 minutes until improvement occurs.
    Rationale:
    α effects cause vasoconstriction and raise B.P.
    β effects cause

Table 17 Catecholamines with varying properties

	β_1	β_2	α	Dopaminergic	Useful dosage range (μg/kg/min)	Indication
Dopamine	+ +	0	+ → + +	+ +	1–5 (loses selectivity at higher doses)	Raises renal perfusion
Dobutamine	+ +	+	+	0	2–40	Positive inotrope
Adrenaline	+ +	+ +	+ → + +	0	0.06–0.18	Anaphylaxis. Cardiac arrest
Isoprenaline	+ +	+ +	0	0	0.02–0.18	Complete heart block (temporising manoeuvre)

(i) bronchodilatation
(ii) reduce mediator release.

1b. i.v. hydrocortisone 300 mg.

2. H₁-antagonist, e.g. chlorpheniramine (Piriton) 10–20 mg slowly i.v.
   Rationale: histamine is one mediator involved — blood histamine
   levels raised in anaphylaxis and correlate with hypotension.

3. General measures:
   raise foot of bed
   volume replacement with i.v. fluids.

4. In severe cases:
   oxygen and possibly intubation and ventilation
   Nebulised β₂-agonist (e.g. salbutamol) for resistant bronchospasm.

HYPERTENSION

Decision to treat hypertension
Based on:
1. Level of BP. At least 3 recordings of raised BP desirable.
2. Evidence of end organ damage: history of cerebral or cardiac
   ischaemia; reduced pulses or vascular bruits; left ventricular
   hypertrophy (by examination, ECG, echocardiogram); impaired
   renal function; severe grades of retinopathy. These all make
   treatment mandatory.
3. Co-existence of other risk factors for vascular disease: smoking;
   hypercholesterolaemia; diabetes mellitus, all favour treatment.
4. Age.
5. Sex.
6. Family history of stroke or sudden death.
7. Evidence of underlying cause (e.g. coarctation,
   phaeochromocytoma) requiring specific treatment.

Treatment of hypertension
A. General
1. Stop smoking.
2. Reduce alchohol consumption if excessive.
3. Reduce salt consumption.
4. Reduce obesity.
5. Treat hyperlipidaemias if present.
6. Regular exercise and relaxation periods.
7. Control diabetes mellitus if present.

B. Specific drug therapy.
No patient is 'routine', each requires consideration of side-effects,
contraindications etc., and the regime is fitted to the patient.
1. Hypertensive encephalopathy — see below.

2. Either a. β-blocker or thiazide diuretic or calcium channel blocker or
   converting enzyme blocker.
   Then b. add β-blocker, thiazide or α_1 blocker (e.g. doxazosin) to
   a. if inadequate response after 6 weeks.
3. For severe hypertension several approaches may need to be tried
   e.g.:
   a. frusemide + β-blocker + minoxidil
   b. diuretic + ACE inhibitor + α_1 blocker.
4. Other drugs such as methyldopa, clonidine may be useful in some
   cases especially when co-existing disease (e.g. asthma, peripheral
   vascular disease, diabetes, gout) contraindicate diuretics and/or
   β-blockers.

Hypertension in pregnancy
Raised diastolic BP associated with slower intra-uterine growth and
increased stillbirth rate.
   Two different types of patient:
1. *Pregnant hypertensives* — higher the BP at mid-term the more
   likely is development of proteinuria and oedema (this may not be
   identical with pre-eclampsia).
2. *Pre-eclampsia* — hypertension in last trimester often accompanied
   by proteinuria and oedema which can progress to eclampsia
   (convulsions, CVA, renal failure, left ventricular failure and
   disseminated intravascular coagulation).

Management
1. Treat diastolic BP > 90–95 mmHg in pregnancy. Longest
   experience with methyldopa but oxprenolol or other β-blockers
   may be as good. Avoid diuretics (ineffective in pregnancy; may
   decrease placental blood flow). ACE inhibitors are absolutely
   contraindicated.
2. Bed rest if above insufficient — allows fetal monitoring. Hydralazine
   can be added to β-blocker treatment. Delivery necessary if control
   impossible.
3. In fulminating hypertension, hydralazine rapidly lowers BP; the
   baby should be delivered as soon as possible.
4. Aspirin may prevent pre-eclampsia in women at risk. This is
   currently under investigation and definite indications are not yet
   clear.

Hypertension in elderly
Treatment of hypertension in healthy elderly individuals is well
worthwhile, provided adverse effects are avoided. Small doses of
diuretics may be effective and well-tolerated; large doses and
complex regimes should be avoided.

β-ADRENOCEPTOR BLOCKING DRUGS
Competitive inhibitors of catecholamine binding at β-adrenoceptors.

Also have other pharmacological properties:
1. Membrane stabilising activity (quinidine-like or local anaesthetic activity).
2. Intrinsic sympathomimetic (partial agonist) activity (ISA) — partially stimulate β-receptor·but prevent effect of natural or exogenous catecholamines.
3. Cardioselectivity: some β-blockers have relatively higher affinity for β_1 (cardiac) adrenergic receptors. These have two *theoretical* advantages:
— may be safer in obstructive airways disease (but should not be used in such patients)
— do not block β_2 (vasodilator) receptors, may be relevant in peripheral vascular disease, hypoglycaemia and possibly hypertension.

Effects of β-blockers

C.V.S.	Reduction of exercise- and anxiety-induced tachycardia
	Negative inotropic action on heart
	Reduction in blood pressure (often delayed)
	Reduced renin release from kidneys
R.S.	Bronchoconstriction in asthmatics
Metabolic	Hypoglycaemia due to reduced gluconeogenesis
C.N.S.	Vivid dreams, confusional states (especially lipid-soluble drugs).
Peripheral nervous system	Reduction of tremor (e.g. due to anxiety, thyrotoxicosis, hypoglycaemia)

Uses of β-blockers
1. Cardiovascular disease:
   hypertension
   angina
   arrhythmias
   post-myocardial infarction (cardioprotective agents) reducing incidence of sudden death
   hypertrophic obstructive cardiomyopathy and Fallot's tetralogy
   phaeochromocytoma (with α-blocker).
2. Nervous system:
   migraine prophylaxis
   essential tremor.
3. Psychiatry:
   anxiety (controls somatic symptoms).
4. Ophthalmology;
   open angle glaucoma (Timolol eye drops — probably decrease aqueous humor formation).
5. Endocrine:
   hyperthyroidism (agents without ISA used to control tachycardia, tremor etc).

Adverse effects of β-blockers
A. *Cardiac*
1. heart failure
2. bradycardia
3. angina and infarction provoked by abrupt withdrawal during treatment of angina.

B. *Peripheral vascular*
Cold extremities, Raynaud's phenomenon.

C. *Pulmonary*
Bronchospasm (in asthmatics).

D. *CNS*
1. nightmares/vivid dreams (especially very lipid soluble drugs like pindolol, propranolol — use atenolol or timolol; avoid evening dose)
2. fatigue — probably partly due to reduced cardiac output
3. impotence.

E. *Diabetes mellitus*
Alters control and reduces awareness of hypoglycaemia.

Contraindications to β-blockers
A. *Cardiac*
1. Absolute
   a. untreated heart failure except some cardiomyopathies (because cardiac output rate-dependent)
   b. heart block/severe bradycardia (β-blockers slow heart further).
2. Relative
   a. treated heart failure (can use β-blockers with diuretics and digitalis)
   b. atypical (Prinzmetal) angina (unopposed α-adrenergic stimulation encourages spasm)
   c. high doses of verapamil (especially i.v.), nifedipine.

B. *Peripheral vascular*
1. Absolute: gangrene (unopposed α-adrenergic effects cause vasoconstriction).
2. Relative: Raynaud's phenomenon; cold extremities; claudication from peripheral vascular disease.

C. *Pulmonary*
1. Absolute: asthma or chronic bronchitis with spasm (unopposed α-adrenergic bronchospasm).
2. Relative: emphysema, acute bronchitis.

Table 18 Vasodilators for chronic administration in hypertension

Drug	Dosage	Pharmacology	Specific adverse effects	Uses
Hydralazine	25 mg 12-hourly up to 300mg/day	Direct acting arterial vasodilator. Subject to polymorphic acetylation. Duration of effect > $T\frac{1}{2}$	S.L.E.-like syndrome (commoner slow acetylators) Peripheral neuropathy (pyridoxine antagonised by metabolite). Serum sickness-like syndrome early in therapy	Pregnancy hypertension
Prazosin	Initially 0.5 mg 12-hourly beginning at night. Increase to max 20 mg/day.	α_1 (post-synaptic) adrenergic blocker. Lowers LDL/HDL ratio	First-dose dizziness or syncope (unusual with low starting dose).	Essential hypertension
Doxazosin	1–16 mg daily starting with a low night-time dose	As prazosin, but long $T\frac{1}{2}$	As prazosin, but first dose hypotension unusual	Essential hypertension
Minoxidil	2.5 mg 12-hourly up to 50 mg/day	Via active sulphone metabolite which activates K^+ channel. Duration of effect > $T\frac{1}{2}$	Excessive hair growth (hypertrichosis) of face, limbs and body. Severe fluid retention	Severe, resistant hypertension
Nifedipine	20 mg 12-hourly — important to specify retard form	Calcium ion antagonist	Flushing, headache, leg swelling	Hypertension
Amlodipine	5–10 mg once daily	As nifedipine but longer $T\frac{1}{2}$	Leg swelling. Less flushing and headaches than nifedipine	Hypertension

D. Diabetes mellitus
Relative: insulin-dependent diabetes.

ACE inhibitors
Captopril enalapril, lisinopril, quinapril, perindopril, fosinopril and ramipril: differ more in price than actions. Fosinopril, enalapril and ramipril are prodrugs.

Pharmacology
Inhibitors of angiotensin converting enzyme (identical with kininase II which breaks down the vasodilator bradykinin). Inhibit the formation of angiotensin II.

Uses
Essential hypertension. Congestive heart failure

Adverse effects
1. Common to all ACE I:
   a. First dose hypotension.
   b. Cough.
   c. Transient taste disturbance.
   d. Renal failure in patients with bilateral renal artery stenosis or in the artery supplying a single functioning kidney.
   e. Hyperkalaemia. This is not usually a disadvantage, but may cause problems in patients with renal impairment especially if they are also receiving $K^{\pm}$ retaining diuretics (e.g. amiloride in Moduretic or Frumil) and/or K^{+} supplements.
   f. Angio-oedema.
2. Associated with −SH groups. These are dose-related and are seldom seen when captopril is used in doses ⩽ 100 mg/day:
   a. Proteinuria and nephrotic syndrome (Paradoxically, small doses of captopril *reduce* proteinuria in diabetics with albuminuria).
   b. Rashes.
   c. Neutropenia.
   d. Myasthenia-like syndrome.

Table 19 Treatment of some hypertensive emergencies

	Drugs	Comments
1. Acute hypertensive encephalopathy	Sodium nitroprusside infusion 1 μg/kg/min up to 8 μg/kg/min	Requires constant monitoring in an ITU with arterial line
2. Accelerated hypertension (grade III or IV fundi without encephalopathy)	Atenolol 50 mg p.o. in first instance. Alternative: methyldopa 250 mg p.o. or nifedipine *retard* 10 mg p.o.	Admit to hospital immediately; avoid i.v. bolus medication; avoid sublingual medication; avoid drugs which cause 1st dose hypotension; avoid diuretics (unless in heart failure)
3. Dissecting aneurysm of aorta	1. Trimetaphan i.v. 2. Sodium nitroprusside infusion (as above) accompanied by β-blockade	Important to reduce dp/dt. ITU monitoring essential. BP lowered until pain disappears provided urinary output maintained. Anatomy defined by radiography and decision for surgery (mainly type 1 and 2) or medical (usually type 3) management made.
4. Phaeochromocytoma	Phenoxybenzamine 10 mg p.o. 12-hourly increased to 40–100 mg 12-hourly as required followed by metoprolol.	Definitive treatment is surgery. Drugs required pre-operatively. α-blockade lowers BP, β-blockade protects heart (NB β-blockers never used alone as unopposed α-effects increase BP). Acute BP crisis treated with phentolamine 5 mg i.v. or by infusion.

11. Drugs acting on the kidneys

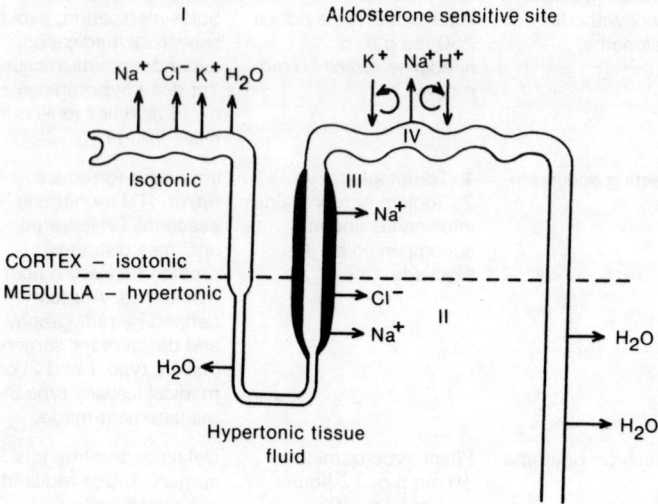

Fig. 11.1

Tubular sites of ionic and water reabsorption
GFR = 180 l/day
Plasma Na^+ conc = 140 mmol/l
so Filtered load of Na^+ = 25 200 mmol/day. Fate of this Na^+:
Site I — removes 67% filtered load
     = 16 800 mmol/day
Site II — removes 25% filtered load
     = 6300 mmol/day
Site III — removes 5% filtered load
     = 1200 mmol/day
Site IV — removes 3% filtered load
     = 750 mmol/day
Urine contains about 0.6% filtered load
     = 150 mmol Na^+/day
Dietary intake of Na^+ = 150 mmol/day to maintain Na^+
homeostasis.

Table 20 Summary of effects of diuretics on sodium reabsorption in the nephron

Diuretic	Glomerular filtration	Zone				% filtered sodium excreted
		I	II	III	IV	
Thiazides	Decreased	Minor inhibition	0	Inhibited	↑ Na$^+$ delivery* increases K$^+$ and H$^+$ loss	5–10
Loop†	Possibly increased	Minor inhibition	Inhibited†	Inhibited	↑ Na$^+$ delivery increases K$^+$ and H$^+$ loss	15–40
Spironolactone Triamterene Amiloride	0	0	0	0	Inhibited (spironolactone competitively blocks action of aldosterone; others are non-competitive inhibitors at this site).	2–5
Carbonic anhydrase inhibitors	0	Weak inhibition	0	0	Weak inhibition	1–2
Osmotic	Possibly increased	0	0	0	↑ Na$^+$ delivery increases K$^+$ and H$^+$ loss	5–10

* also reduce the permeability of tubules to water and hence relieve diabetes insipidus
† primary action is powerful inhibition of chloride reabsorption in Zone II (ascending limb of the loop of Henle).

THIAZIDES AND RELATED DRUGS

Actions

All have similar actions — but the more water-soluble ones are shorter-acting as they have a lower V_d and more rapid elimination. High protein binding — correlates with increasing duration of action.

1. Diuresis mainly by action on Zone III (inhibit Na^+, K^+-ATPase and limit energy available for transport) reducing Cl^- reabsorption
   Also inhibition of carbonic anhydrase
   Stimulation of K^+/Na^+ exchange at Zone IV (therefore K^+ loss)
2. Hypotension due to vasodilation and Na^+ loss.
3. Thiazides also produce antidiuresis in diabetus insipidus patients: possibly by reduction in GFR and/or reduction in thirst and/or increase permeability of tubules to water.
4. Reduction in Ca^{++} excretion useful in idiopathic hypercalciuria.

Uses

1. Generalised and localised oedema (e.g. heart failure, nephrotic syndrome).
2. Hypertension.
3. Diabetes insipidus.
4. Reduction of urinary stone formation in idiopathic hypercalciuria.

Adverse effects

1. Hypokalaemia (also Mg^{++} lost in urine). Potassium loss can precipitate coma in patients with cirrhosis.
2. Impaired glucose tolerance — about 10% after 6 years chronic therapy.
3. Hyperuricaemia — can precipitate acute gout.
4. Consequences of diuresis, e.g. hyponatraemia; urinary retention in men with prostatic hypertrophy.
5. Impotence.
6. Effects of uncertain significance: Elevation of plasma renin, cholesterol and reduction of high density lipoproteins.
7. Uncommon: allergy (and light sensitivity); thrombocytopenia (rarely other blood dyserasias); pancreatitis; hypercalcaemia.
8. Interactions: reduced lithium clearance predisoposing to toxicity; potentiates skeletal muscle relaxants.

Bendrofluazide 2.5 mg has an antihypertensive effect with little biochemical disturbance. Larger doses are used in heart failure.

Chlorthalidone has a more prolonged action.

Metazolone has a powerful diuretic action when given with a loop diuretic.

Xipamide is the most powerful thiazide diuretic.

Indapamide lowers blood pressure with little diabetogenic or other metabolic actions.

LOOP (HIGH CEILING) DIURETICS

Produce a very powerful diuresis even in the face of a low GFR. Unlike thiazides increasing dose increases effect over a wide range (hence called high-ceiling).

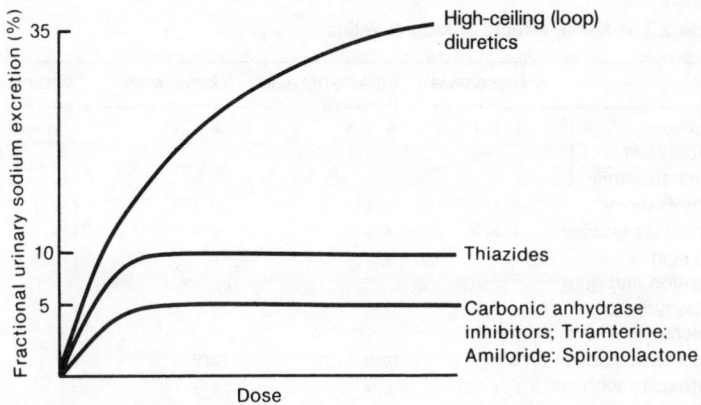

Fig. 11.2 Dose-response curves (diagrammatic) for diuretics.

Loop diuretics

Approved name		Start of diuresis	Duration of action
Frusemide	oral	30 mins	6 h
	i.v.	10 mins	6 h
Ethacrynic acid	oral	30 mins	6 h
	i.v.	10 mins	6 h
Bumetanide	oral	20 mins	4–6 h
	i.v.	5–10 mins	4–6 h
Piretanide	Not used as a diuretic, but is antihypertensive		

NB
1. All loop diuretics can produce hyponatraemia (without reduced total body Na^+) due to 'inappropriate' ADH secretion in response to stimulus of reduced ECF volume. Treat by water restriction.

2. Frusemide potentiates renal toxicity of cephaloridine and ototoxicity of gentamicin.
3. Actions of frusemide antagonised by indomethacin, aspirin.

Uses
1. Generalized/localised oedema unresponsive to thiazides.
2. Pulmonary oedema — frusemide has powerful vasodilator action which accounts in part for effectiveness.
3. Natriuresis in renal failure.
4. Hypercalcaemia (frusemide).

Table 22 Adverse effects of loop diuretics

	Frusemide	Ethacrynic acid	Bumetanide	Piretanide
Acute hypovolaemia Hyponatraemia	+ + +	+ + +	+ + +	+ + +
K⁺ deficiency	+ + +	+ + +	+ + +	+ + +
Ca⁺⁺ loss in urine	+ +	+ +	+ +	+ +
Uric acid retention and gout	+	+	+	+
Carbohydrate intolerance	+	+	+	+
Blood dyscrasias	rare	rare	rare	?
Ototoxicity with high doses	+ +	+ +	+ +	?
Muscle pain	0	0	+	+
GI toxicity	+	+ + +	+	+

0 = absent
$+$ = mild or low risk
$+ +$ = moderate
$+ + +$ = considerable

CARBONIC ANHYDRASE INHIBITORS (See Fig. 11.3)

ACETAZOLAMIDE
Inhibits carbonic anhydrase in eyes, brain and kidney; weak diuretic, action terminated by acidosis produced by the drug.

Uses
1. Narrow angle glaucoma: i.v. 250–500 mg in acute cases followed by 250 mg orally 6-hourly (sustained release tabs — Sustets — given twice daily).
2. Cysteine renal calculi.
3. Prophylaxis of mountain sickness.
4. Rarely for epilepsy in childhood.
5. Periodic paralysis (both hyperkalaemic and hypokalaemic varieties).

Table 23 Potassium sparing diuretics

Drug	Duration of action	Special properties
Spironolactone (canrenone is active metabolite) ⎫ Potassium canrenoate (metabolised to canrenone) ⎭	10 h	Useful in oedema of cirrhosis and severe heart failure Can produce: hyperkalaemia nausea hirsutes gynaecomastia menstrual irregularity abolishes activity of carbenoxelone large doses: ataxia, confusion
Amiloride	6 h ⎫	Weak diuretics Can produce potassium retention Given with thiazides or loop diuretics as an alternative to giving potassium supplements
Triameterine	2 h ⎭	

6. Reduction of intracranial hypertension (reduces CSF formation).

Adverse effects
1. Paraesthesia, fatigue, somnolence, malaise.
2. Dyspepsia, substernal burning.
3. Hypersensitivity and blood dyscrasias.

OSMOTIC DIURETICS

MANNITOL
Administered i.v as a 10 or 20% solution for:
1. accelerating elimination of poisons
2. impending renal failure
3. reduction of intraocular pressure ⎰ i.v. urea or glycerol
4. reduction of intracerebral pressure ⎱ alternative osmotic diuretics

Adverse effects
1. Increase in plasma volume may precipitate heart failure.
2. Potassium loss.

POTASSIUM AND DIURETICS

Serum K^+ is unreliable indicator of total body K^+ (98% of body's 3500 mM is intracellular). Acid-base changes also disturb extra/intra cellular balance.

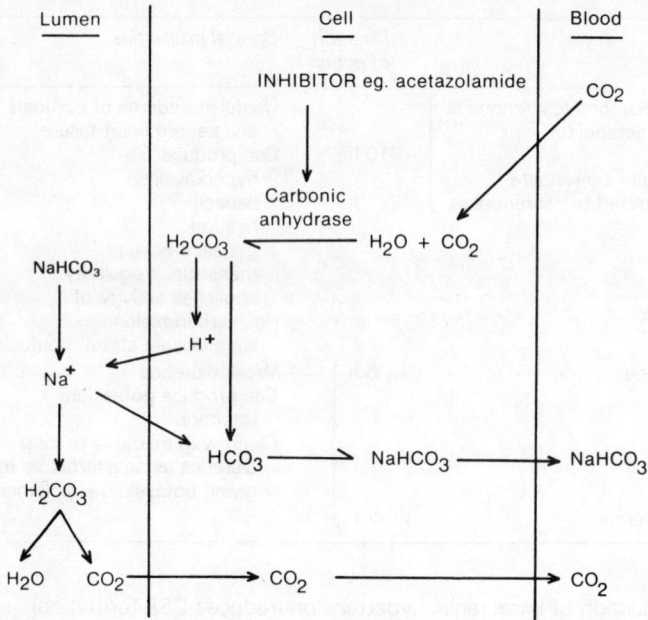

Fig. 11.3

In practie if levels < 3 mmol/l a significant K^+ deficit (up to 400 mM) is assumed. This needs treatment to prevent cardiac arrhythmias, ileus, nephropathy, muscle weakness and potentiation of digitalis toxicity.

K^+ status of all patients on diuretics ($\pm$ K^+ supplements) requires monitoring at least pre-treatment, after 3 months diuretics and then yearly.

Hypokalaemia following diuretic therapy
Diuretic therapy produces initial fall in serum K^+ within 1–2 weeks of starting treatment — but new steady-state then established and progressive deficit does not occur. Up to 50% of hypertensives on thiazides have serum K^+ between 3.0 and 3.5 mmol/l (represents 5–10% reduction in total body K^+). Less than 10% of patients have serum K^+ < 3.0 mmol/l;. In patients with mild heart failure on frusemide corresponding figures are 5% <3.5 mmol/l and 0.2% <3.0 mmol/l. Average fall in serum K^+ is 0.6 mmol/l after thiazides; 0.3 mmol/l after 40–80 mg frusemide.

Patients with hypertension or mild heart failure exhibit similar falls in serum K^+ but in heart failure initial levels are higher and the incidence of hypokalaemia is decreased.

Measures to reduce potassium loss

Patients with heart failure — small doses of loop diuretics waste less potassium than thiazides.

Patients with hypertension — doses of thiazides as low as 5 mg bendrofluazide produce near maximal effects.

Moderate salt restriction (to 70–80 mM daily) — no added salt and avoidance of salty foods — lowers diuretic requirements and reduces renal potassium losses.

Dietary measures — additional meat and fish expensive but potassium rich foods also include milk, potatoes, carrots, parsnips, tomatoes, celery, leeks, dried fruits, nuts, bananas, rhubarb and soft fruits.

Indications for potassium replacement

Provided no contraindications (e.g. renal impairment) *prophylactic potassium* replacement needed in the following 'high risk' situations:

High doses of diuretics.

Concurrent digoxin, acute myocardial infarction or serious heart disease.

Concurrent drugs altering ventricular repolarisation (phenothiazines, tricyclic antidepressants).

Hyperaldosteronism
— severe congestive cardic failure
— severe liver disease, e.g. cirrhosis (hypokalaemia precipitates coma)
— nephrotic syndrome.

Concurrent potassium-losing therapy
— corticosteroids and ACTH
— carbenoxolone
— laxatives.

Poor K^+ intake — usually elderly (check renal function).

Pre-treatment potassium level <3.5 mmol/l.

Serum potassium levels falling below 3.0 mmol/l require *correction*.

Potassium replacement

Potassium supplements

Limited effect in the prevention of diuretic-induced hypokalaemia. 24–48 mmol/day is needed and correction of hypokalaemia may require more. As most preparations contain 8–12 mmol, daily doses of at least 3–6 tablets can cause problems with compliance.

Combined diuretic/potassium tablets (contain only 7–8 mmol K^+) may be inadequate.

KCl preferred as corrects hypochloraemia and alkalosis associated with hypokalaemia.

Adverse effects

Nausea, vomiting, diarrhoea, abdominal discomfort, bad taste. Risk of ulceration if GI transit delay: can cause scarring of oesophagus and duodenum.

Drugs producing salt and water retention
Results in oedema; hypertension; increased cardiac failure.
1. Corticosteroids and ACTH (occasionally anabolic steroids).
2. Oestrogens.
3. Non-steroidal anti-inflammatory drugs, e.g. phenylbutazone.
4. Carbenoxolone.
5. Arterial vasodilators, e.g. hydralazine, minoxidil.
6. Sometimes other antihypertensive agents in particular guanethidine, methyldopa.
7. Lithium.

Drugs containing unexpectedly large amounts of sodium
1. Antacids — some, e.g. Gaviscon, aluminium hydroxide gel — also over the counter preparations, e.g. Andrew's Liver Salts.
2. Penicillins — large doses given i.v., e.g. carbenicillin sodium.
3. X-ray contrast media, e.g. Conray.

Treatment for ascites
1. Salt and water restriction — mild cases Na intake <22 mmol/day (0.5 g); severe cases <10 mmol/day. Diets unpalatable.
2. Diuretics — spironolactone (counteracts hyperaldosteronism) but slow and care needed if renal impairment. Add frusemide if no effect after few days on 100 mg 6-hourly. Thiazides also used with spironolactone.
3. Bed rest (but look out for DVTs!).
   Aim for loss of no more 1000 ml/day (best judged by body weight) since mobilisation of oedema fluid is slow and greater diuresis 'shrinks' plasma volume and is dangerous.
   Resistant cases try:
1. Infusion of salt-poor albumin (not more than 50 g) with large dose diuretic if severe hypoalbuminaemia present. Maintain albumin around 40 g/l if possible.
2. Corticosteroids may produce effect if given for up to a week (? mechanism).
3. Mannitol.
4. Rarely haemodialysis.

Management of gravitational oedema
1. Diuretics — alone do not control postural oedema.
2. Mobilise.
3. Support legs with elastic stockings.
4. Isometric exercises especially for chair-bound.
5. Elevate foot of bed and feet when seated.
6. Treat heart failure, hypoalbuminaemia, anaemia.

Anaemia. The anaemia of chronic renal failure can be significantly improved by giving recombinant erythropoietin.

ALTERATION OF URINARY pH

1. To increase drug elimination in overdose

Principle
Non-ionised drug equilibrates rapidly across membranes and can be reabsorbed from renal tubule into blood.
Ionised drug cannot be reabsorbed.
Thus adjusting urinary pH to promote drug ionisation increases urinary drug excretion.

Henderson-Hasselbalch equation:

$$pH = pK_a + \log \frac{[A^-]}{[HA]}$$

$$[A^-] = H^+ \text{ acceptor}; [HA] = H^+ \text{ donor}$$

so

$$\log \frac{[A^-]}{[HA]} = pH - pK_a$$

NB
a. If $pH = pK_a$ both acids and bases are 50 per cent ionised.
b. Acids are more ionised when $pH > pK_a$.
   Bases are more ionised when $pH < pK_a$.

Example
Phenobarbitone pK_a 7.3.

Urine	Plasma	Urine
pH 5.3	pH 7.3	pH 8.3
$\log \frac{[A^-]}{[HA]} = 5.3 - 7.3$	$\log \frac{[A^-]}{[HA]} = 7.3 - 7.3$	$\log \frac{[A^-]}{[HA]} = 8.3 - 7.3$
$= -2$	$= 0$	$= 1$
$\frac{[A^-]}{[HA]} = 10^{-2}$	$\frac{[A^-]}{[HA]} = 1$	$\frac{[A^-]}{[HA]} = 10$
$= \frac{0.01}{1}$	$= \frac{1}{1}$	$= \frac{10}{1}$

Conclusion: The proportion of ionised (and therefore non-reabsortion) phenobarbitone increases 1000 fold by changing urinary pH from 5.3 to 8.3.

Drugs whose elimination is usefully promoted by manipulation of urinary pH:

Alkaline diuresis	Acid diuresis
Barbitone	Amphetamine
Phenobarbitone	Pethidine
Salicylate	

NB Most barbiturates are eliminated by metabolism and are not amenable to forced alkaline diuresis.

2. To increase efficacy of antimicrobials in urine.

Acid	Alkali
Tetracycline	Streptomycin
Penicillin	Sulphonamides

3. To discourage growth of certain urinary pathogens, e.g. *E. coli* (alkaline).

4. Symptomatic relief of 'cystitis'.

5. To render drugs or metabolites more soluble to prevent crystalluria (e.g. sulphonamides-alkaline) or stone formation (e.g. urate-alkaline).

Drugs for alkalinisation
1. i.v. or oral sodium bicarbonate.
2. i.v. sodium lactate (converted to bicarbonate in vivo).
3. Oral sodium or potassium citrate.

Drugs for acidification
1. Oral ammonium chloride (converted to ammonia ($\rightarrow$ urea) and HCl).
2. Oral methionine (converted to equivalent of H_2SO_4).
3. Oral arginine hydrochloride (equivalent to HCl).
4. Oral or i.v. ascorbic acid.

12. Drugs acting on the respiratory system

ASTHMA

Asthma: a condition of airways obstruction which (in the earlier stages of the disease at least) is reversible.

Obstruction due to:
1. smooth muscle contraction
2. inflammation of the airway wall
3. plugging with viscid mucus and leucocytes.

Therapeutic agents are divided into:
1. Bronchodilators: β-agonists anticholinergics theophylline
2. Anti-inflammatory/prophylactic: glucocorticoids, sodium cromoglycate and nedocromil sodium.

β-AGONISTS

All can induce tremor (β$_2$ actions) and may produce tachycardia secondary to vasodilatation. β-agonists raise intracellular cAMP.

GLUCOCORTICOIDS

Anti-inflammatory glucocorticoids are effective in chronic asthma when they are usually given by inhalation. Oral and intravenous glucocorticoids are important in the treatment of acute asthma.

OTHER PROPHYLACTIC DRUGS
Sodium cromoglycate (SCG; Intal)
Reduces local cholinergic reflexes and may have mast cell stabilising activity.

Administration
1. Metered aerosol 5 mg/puff. Dose is 2 puffs 6-hourly.
2. Nebuliser solution 10 mg/ml; 20 mg nebulised 4–6 times daily. Can be used in young children.
3. As Spincaps (20 mg) inhaled as a powder using a Spinhaler.
Pharmacokinetics. Not absorbed from gut.
Toxicity. Hoarseness and mild wheezing. Bronchospasm can be precipitated, but this is rare.

Table 24(a) β-agonist drugs in asthma

Drug	Administration	Selectivity	Clinical properties
Salbutamol	Aerosol 100 μg/dose. Rotacaps 400 μg Oral 2–4 mg 6-hourly. Oral sustained release 4–8 mg. i.v 4 μg/kg by slow injection. s.c. and i.m. 8 μg/kg. 5 mg/ml solution for inhalation	Selective β₂-agonist. (Equieffective β₂ action to isoprenaline with 1/10 of β₁ effect)	No hepatic or pulmonary 1st pass metabolism, $T^{1/2}$ = 2–4 h. Can produce tremor and mild tachycardia. Leg cramps at night are common
Terbutaline	Aerosol 250 μg/dose; dry powder. Turbohaler 500 μg/dose Oral 5 mg 8–12 hourly. 10 mg/ml solution for inhalation via nebuliser	Selective β₂-agonist (twice bronchodilator action of isoprenaline with ¼ of cardiostimulatory effect)	Small degree of 1st pass metabolism (sulphatation by gut wall) but effective orally. Not metabolised when given i.v. $T^{1/2}$ = 3–4 h
Rimiterol	Aerosol 200 μg/dose. Can be given i.v.	Selective β₂-agonist (similar to salbutamol when given i.v. but similar to isoprenaline inhaled)	$T^{1/2}$ approx 2 h
Fenoterol	Aerosol 100–200 μg/dose 2 or 3 times daily	Selective β₂-agonist (similar to salbutamol, but may have more cardiac stimulation)	Similar properties to salbutamol but longer acting $T^{1/2}$ = 7h
Salmeterol	Aerosol or diskhaler 50 μg 12 hourly	Same as salbutamol	Prolonged action with bronchodilatation and protection against challenge for up to 12 hours. Useful in nocturnal asthma

Table 24(b) Glucocorticoids used in asthma

Drug	Dose	Properties
Cortisol (Hydrocortisone)	Initial i.v. dose of 4 mg/kg of hemisuccinate, followed by 6 hourly doses of 3 mg/kg or continuous infusion of 3 mg/kg 6-hourly	Subjective improvement in 1–4 hours, objective improvement from 6 h after first dose. (Plasma levels of cortisol of 100 µg/100 ml needed for optimum response.)
Prednisolone	In acute asthma 40 mg immediately , then 20 mg 6 hourly for 24 hours, then 30–40 mg daily. In deteriorating asthma 20–30 mg daily for 7–14 days. If used in chronic asthma, give the smallest effective dose	Similar properties to cortisol (but 4–5 × anti-inflammatory with same mineralocorticoid effects)
Beclomethasone dipropionate	Various types and strengths of inhaler, 50–250 µg per inhalation as metered dose inhalers, Rotacaps, Diskhaler. 400–2000 µg/day usually as 2 divided doses. Also given via a spacing device (1000 µg or more) and, by nebuliser (for children)	Powerful anti-inflammatory actions — little is absorbed systemically from lungs. Suppression of pituitary-adrenal axis. Around 1600 µg/day. Candidiasis of mouth in 5% of patients. Hoarseness occasionally
Betamethasone valerate	400 µg as daily dose (divided) from metered aerosol	
Budenoside	400–2000 µg/day as 2 divided doses	Similar to beclomethasone

Nedocromil sodium is another prophylactic for adults with asthma. It powerfully inhibits the release of mediators from lung mast cells *in vitro*. It is effective in preventing attacks precipitated by antigens, exercise, cold and sulphur dioxide. It is administered from a pressurised aerosol dispenser.

Ketotifen

Pharmacokinetics and action
Absorbed from gut. In addition to mast cell stabilisation, blocks histamine H_1 receptors (and has anticholinergic and sedative actions). Little, if any, place in routine treatment.

Toxicity.   Sedation, dry mouth. Drying of bronchial secretions may aggravate asthma.

METHYL XANTHINES

Only theophylline and its derivatives are widely used members of this group. Aminophylline is theophylline with ethylene diamine.

Administration
Oral: many forms, e.g. choline theophylline, sustained release aminophylline
Rectal: aminophylline suppositories.
i.v.: aminophylline given by *slow* infusion over at least 15 minutes as a loading dose followed by a lower strength infusion. In patients already taking oral theophylline, the loading dose should be adjusted according to the blood level. If this is not available the loading dose should be halved or omitted.

Pharmacokinetics
Absorbed well from small intestine. $T\frac{1}{2}$ = 3–10 h; elimination mainly by hepatic metabolism and 10% excreted unchanged in urine. Rectally it causes local irritation, and absorption is erratic. Reduced clearance in infants under 6 months, acutely ill adults with cirrhosis, cardiac failure, cor pulmonale. Increased clearance in smokers and in patients taking rifampicin. Clearance is reduced by erythromycin, ciprofloxacin and cimetidine.

Effective plasma level
8–20 µg/ml.

Toxic effects
Nausea, vomiting
Tachycardia, cardiac arrhythmias
Hyperventilation
Insomnia, anxiety, headache, fits

Enprofylline is a xanthine which is not a phosphodiesterase inhibitor. It is a powerful bronchodilator, but does not show CNS and cardiac toxicity.

Anticholinergics (ipratropium bromide and oxitropium bromide) are given by inhalation of a metered aerosol. Ipratropium is available as a nebuliser solution. In older patients the effects may be more than β–agonists. Oxitropium has a more prolonged action.

DRUG TREATMENT OF ASTHMA

Control of asthma should be monitored with peak flow recording at home using mini peak flow meters, particularly during times of change in treatment.

A. Chronic asthma

In chronic asthma, drugs should be given by the inhaled route whenever possible. This minimises toxic effects. Technique must be checked but there are enough types of inhaler to allow most patients to use this route.

1. Bronchodilators should be used for symptomatic relief of airflow obstruction. β_2 agonists (such as salbutamol) are most useful. They should be given by the inhaled route — this can be used by children down to 3 or 4 years with dry powder inhalers or spacer devices. Bronchodilators can also be used to prevent asthma, such as before exercise. When the bronchodilator response is inadequate, higher doses or addition of an anticholinergic such as ipratropium bromide may be helpful.

2. When bronchodilators are needed one or more times a day, then prophylactic drugs should be considered. Sodium cromoglycate may be effective in mild asthma and in childhood. A 6-week trial should be given to assess its effectiveness. Inhaled corticosteroids should be used in more severe asthma or when sodium cromoglycate does not give adequate control. The steroid may be given with bronchodilators and the dose adjusted according to response.

3. Airway calibre in asthma shows a diurnal variation with lowest peak flows in the early hours of the morning. Nocturnal symptoms are often reduced by inhaled corticosteroids, but if symptoms persist then long acting bronchodilators such as inhaled salmeterol or oral slow release theophylline may be necessary.

4. When symptoms or peak flow records show deteriorating asthma, a 10–14 day course of oral corticosteroids may prevent a severe attack and re-establish control.

B. Acute severe asthma

1. Sedatives and opioids are contraindicated.

2. If the patient's usual β-agonist aerosol is ineffective then arrange to admit to hospital. While waiting for the ambulance give oxygen if available and salbutamol by nebuliser or subcutaneous injection; also 300 mg of cortisol i.v. (as succinate or hemisuccinate) or 60 mg oral prednisolone.

In hospital

3. Steroids take several hours to act and early relief relies on bronchodilators:
   a) Salbutamol 2.5–5 mg is given by nebuliser driven by oxygen and the patient reassessed after 10–15 minutes. If the response is inadequate then nebulisation should be repeated with the addition of 500 µg ipratropium bromide. The treatment can be repeated at 1–4 hour intervals.
   b) If nebuliser treatment fails intravenous bronchodilators can be given either as an infusion of salbutamol 5–15 µg/kg/h or

aminophylline given (slowly) as a loading infusion followed by a lower dose infusion.

c) In severe asthma intravenous hydrocortisone is given 300 mg initially then 200 mg 6-hourly. In less severe disease 40 mg of oral prednisolone is given initially followed by 20 mg 6-hourly. After 24–48 hours the dose of steroid can usually be reduced to 30–40 mg prednisolone daily.

d) Blood gases should be measured and oxygen given by MC mask. In older patients with chronic airflow obstruction and a raised Pa_{co_2} on presentation, the inspired oxygen should be controlled at 24–28% by Ventimask.

e) If there is dehydration, fluid is given. Potassium levels should be measured and potassium given as necessary.

f) When a bacterial infection has precipitated the attack, an antibiotic such as amoxycillin or erythromycin should be given.

g) When treatment is failing and the patient tiring or blood gases deteriorating then ventilatory support is considered.

h) It is essential that every acute attack should lead to an investigation of the patient's regular treatment and the reason for loss of control.

COMMON COLD

Very little can be done. 0.5–1 g of ascorbic acid may reduce the severity and possibly shorten the course of the disease. Proprietary mixtures containing antihistamines and various analgesics and vasoconstrictors may also alleviate some of the symptoms.

ALLERGIC RHINITIS

Non sedating H_1 antihistamines (terfenadine, astemizole, acrivastine, cetirizine and loratidine) may be helpful. Topical steroids (beclomethasone, flunisolide and budesonide) given as nasal aerosol. Cromoglycate eye drops or ointment effective in allergic conjunctivitis.

Nasal ipratropium may control the watery rhinorrhoea in perennial rhinitis.

Topical steroids should be started before the pollen season and continued regularly while further exposure to pollen, or other precipitants, is likely.

ACUTE BRONCHITIS

No benefit (but possible harm) from antibiotics in otherwise fit persons, but serious deterioration can be prevented if they are used in patients with underlying lung disease.

CHRONIC BRONCHITIS AND EMPHYSEMA (CHRONIC OBTRUCTIVE LUNG DISEASE; 'COLD')

Much of the damage is irreversible by the time of presentation. Prevention by stopping tobacco smoking is the most important aspect of management.

1. Stop smoking; avoid cold and damp atmospheres; avoid irritating pollutants.
2. Treat acute exacerbations due to bacterial infections with chemotherapy: amoxycillin produces double the sputum concentration of same dose of ampicillin; tetracycline effective in bacterial and mycoplasmal infections and penetrates sputum adequately at a dose of 500 mg 6-hourly. Doxycycline (200 mg stat and 100 mg daily) also effective and can be used in renal insufficiency. Cotrimoxazole (2 tablets, 12 hourly) effective but sulphamethoxazole penetrates sputum poorly.
3. Improve sputum removal with exercise and postural drainage.
4. Prevent exacerbations, e.g. amantadine; influenza immunisation; pneumococcal vaccine; antibacterials at first sign of a cold; avoid outdoor work in bad weather.
5. It is very important to treat airways obstruction although in such patients complete reversal is unlikely. However, valuable responses can be achieved. Inhaled bronchodilators are given and responses assessed subjectively and by peak flow measurements. Anticholinergics may produce better responses than β_2 agonists in some older patients. When obstruction is severe a two week trial of oral corticosteroids will establish how much reversibility is achievable and whether long term inhaled corticosteroids should be used.
6. When a Pa_{O_2} in a stable situation is less than 6.9 kPa on two occasions and can be raised to 8 kPa without CO_2 retention then long term home oxygen is considered. This has been shown to reduce mortality and morbidity when used more than 15 h daily, and the closer to 24 h use the better. This can be provided at home by an oxygen concentrator.
7. Adequate nutrition and reduction of excess weight are important factors in long term management.

RESPIRATORY FAILURE

Defined as Pa_{O_2} < 8 kPa (< 60 mmHg) with or without Pa_{CO_2} > 6.3 kPa (> 47 mmHg)

Type I Ventilation/perfusion inequality (pneumonia, LVF, pulmonary fibrosis, shock lung) gives a normal or lowered Pa_{CO_2}.

Type II Respiration depression or severe ventilation/perfusion inequality in chronic bronchitis and emphysema gives increased Pa_{CO_2} with low Pa_{O_2}.

Treatment
1. Treat the underlying disease, e.g. antibiotics in pneumonia, bronchodilators and steroids in airflow obstruction.
2. Oxygen. High inspired oxygen in type I respiratory failure. In type II respiratory failure oxygen can be given freely in respiratory depression but ventilatory support or drug antagonists (naloxone for opioids and flumazenil for benzodiazepines) may be necessary. In chronic airflow obstruction controlled oxygen, 24% or 28%, by Ventimask. If this provokes CO_2 retention, then the respiratory stimulant, doxapram may be given during oxygen administration. However artificial ventilation should be considered. Whether to embark on ventilatory support may be a difficult decision in patients with severe chronic respiratory disease.

13. Drugs for gastrointestinal disease

ANTIEMETICS

Different emetic mechanisms involved in different cases.
Anticholinergic drugs useful in motion sickness (acting on vestibular nuclei and vomiting centre). Phenothiazines and metoclopramide (act mainly on chemoreceptor trigger zone) have little effect on motion sickness, but are effective in vomiting caused by anticancer drugs.

Vomiting in pregnancy treated if possible by diet and reassurance regarding its self-limiting nature. Drugs may be held responsible for fetal malformation, and therefore ideally no drugs should be given in the first trimester. Evidence for antiemetic teratogenicity is minimal. Meclozine as Ancoloxin (meclozine HCl 25 mg; pyridoxine HCl 50 mg) given as 2 tablets at bedtime has been used for many years. Prochlorperazine is used in severe vomiting in pregnancy.

Antiemetics include:
1. metoclopramide and domperidone
2. anticholinergics
3. antihistamines
4. neuroleptics
5. betahistine (for Ménière's disease only)
6. cannabinoids, e.g. nabilone
7. steroids
8. $5HT_3$ antagonists.

METOCLOPRAMIDE

Pharmacology
Derivative of procainamide.
1. Blocks central dopaminergic receptors. Is antiemetic by inhibiting chemoreceptor trigger zone. Extrapyramidal syndromes may be induced.
2. Sensitises gut muscle to acetylcholine and releases acetylcholine from cholinergic nerves in gut; little effect on other cholinergic mechanisms. Possible action of gastric dopamine receptors.
   Actions on gut include:
   a. increased tone of lower oesophageal sphincter

b. increased contraction of oesophagus, antrum and small intestine
c. relaxation of pylorus.

Uses
1. Antiemetic, e.g. in anaesthesia, cancer chemotherapy, radiation sickness.
2. Gastro-oesophageal reflux and oesophagitis.

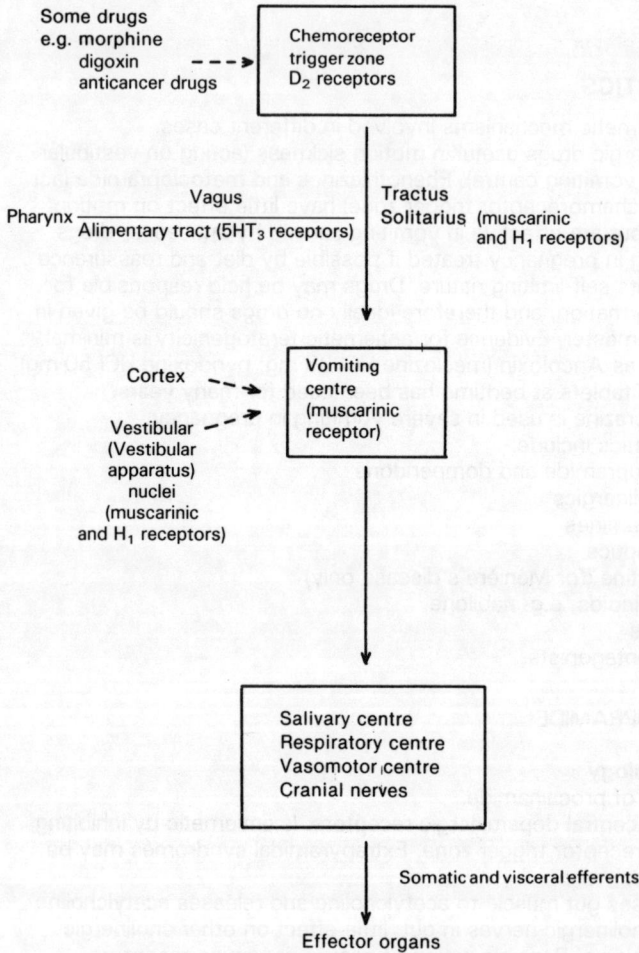

Fig. 13.1 Emetic pathways (putative transmitter shown in brackets).

3. Diagnostic radiography and intubation.
4. Gastric motor failure.
5. To improve analgesic absorption in migraine attacks.

Adverse effects
Dizziness and faintness
Extrapyramidal syndromes — akathisia, dystonia; oculogyric crises,
torticollis, facial spasms (commoner in young)
Tardive dyskinesias (commoner in the old).

Domperidone. Similar to metoclopramide but less CNS penetration,
thus less extrapyramidal toxicity. However dyskinesis and tardive
dyskinesias may be caused.
Intravenously can precipitate cardiac arrhythmias.

Nabilone (Cesamet). A synthetic cannabinoid used with cytotoxic
therapy only. Given orally. Toxicity includes dysphoria, sedation and
dizzyness. Acts on chemoreceptor trigger zone.

Ondansetron. This is valuable in treating nausea and vomiting in
patients receiving cytotoxic drugs or radiotherapy who have not
responded to other antiemetics. Toxic effects include constipation,
headache and sensations of warmth over the head and abdomen.
    It acts as a 5-HT antagonist on $5-HT_3$ receptors.

OESOPHAGEAL DISORDERS

LESP (lower oesophageal sphincter pressure) most important factor in
controlling gastro-oesophageal reflux.

Drug effects on LESP

Increased LESP	Decreased LESP
Antacids	Nicotine
	Caffeine
Metoclopramide	Nitrates
Cholinergic drugs	Anticholinergic drugs
Protein meals	Fatty meals

1. Reflux oesophagitis
May occur in absence of anatomical hiatus hernia.
   a. General advice: reduce weight; raise head of bed (but not to
      sleep with more pillows which raises intra-abdominal pressure);
      avoid stooping and abdominal constriction; stop smoking;
      reduce size of evening meal; no alcohol taken in the evening.
   b. Antacids ± polymethylsiloxane or alginate preparations to
      relieve flatulence and pain. Used after meals and at bed-time.

Table 25 Some antiemetic drugs

Drug	Mode of action	Toxicity	Uses
Anticholinergics: hyoscine	Antimuscarinic action on the gut and central inhibition of vomiting centre	Drowsiness Dry mouth Blurred vision Urinary retention	Preoperative medication, motion sickness, labyrinthitis, Ménière's disease
Antihistamines: cyclizine dimenhydrinate promethazine cinnarizine	Antimuscarinic and antihistamine (H_1) actions on vestibular nuclei and tractus solitarius	Drowsiness Dry mouth Blurred vision	Motion sickness and other forms of labyrinthine vomiting
Neuroleptics: chlorpromazine prochlorperazine perphenazine methotrimeprazine droperidol	Block dopamine (D_2) receptors in chemoreceptor zone	Postural hypotension Extrapyramidal effects	Postoperative, post radiation, drug induced vomiting
Betahistine (Serc)	Partial agonist of histamine — exerts vasodilatation like histamine, but can relieve histamine headache	Aggravation of asthma and peptic ulcer. Can produce nausea. Contraindicated in phaeochromocytoma	Vertigo and nausea in Ménière's disease.

c. *Metoclopramide* 30 mins before meals aids gastric emptying and increased LESP.

Cisapride stimulates gastric motility and reduces reflux by promoting acetylcholine release. It can cause abdominal cramps and diarrhroea.

d. H_2 antagonists: reduce acidity and reduce erosive oesophagitis. NB Anticholinergic drugs contraindicated.

2. Diffuse oesophageal spasm
Nitrates, e.g. nitroglycerine, or long-acting erythritol tetranitrate sometimes used for pain and dysphagia.

MANAGEMENT OF PEPTIC ULCER
A. General
1. Bed rest — heals G.U., may symptomatically improve D.U.
2. Stop smoking.
3. Diet — food acts as antacid so frequent small meals help symptoms.
4. Avoid 'irritants', e.g. caffeine, alcohol, NSAID.

B. Drugs
Remember disappearance of symptoms does not prove ulcer healed. Endoscopy ensures accurate diagnosis and excludes carcinoma of the stomach.

H_2blockers, sucralfate, bismuth chelate, pirenzepine, misoprostol or carbenoxelone for initial therapy. Antacids are used symptomatically. Resistant ulcers usually respond to the proton pump inhibitor omeprazole. Recurrent ulcers may be treated with bismuth plus antibacterials.

H_2 BLOCKERS
CIMETIDINE

Actions
Prevents gastrin, vagal stimulation and histamine from enhancing gastric acid secretion by competitive antagonism of histamine at H_2-receptor. Volume of acid secreted is reduced and pepsin secretion secondarily decreased. No effect on intrinsic factor secretion or gut motility. No rebound increase in gastric acid secretion when treatment stopped. Probably effective when given at night only.

Clinical uses
1. Duodenal ulcers.
2. Gastric ulcers — evidence for efficacy in lesser curve and proximal ulcers less convincing than for pyloric and preplyoric ulcers.
3. Postoperative stomal ulcers.
4. Peptic oesophagitis.

5. Zollinger-Ellison syndrome.
6. Prevention of upper GI bleeding after burns, trauma, acute renal failure etc.
7. Prevention of acid inactivation of pancreatic extracts (enzymes) in pancreatic insufficiency.
8. No good evidence of efficacy in established GI bleeding or in acute gastritis.
9. Reduces liver blood flow in portal hypertension and bleeding oesophageal varices.

NB Malignant gastric ulcers may symptomatically respond: exclusion of malignancy is mandatory before cimetidine treatment.

Adverse effects

Usually well tolerated — minor effects include diarrhoea, dizziness, myalgia and rashes.

Stomach — No evidence of carcinogenesis in man.

CVS — Cardiac arrhythmias (bradycardia, A–V dissociation) are very rare. Rapid i.v. injection rarely causes hypotension.

CNS — Reversible confusional states, hallucinations, drowsiness tremor and dizziness can occur usually but not necessarily in elderly or in renal failure.

Endocrine — Breast tenderness, gynaecomastia and galactorrhoea (? direct action on breast tissue, ?? hyperprolactinaemia).

Anti-androgenic: loss of libido, erectile impotence, reduced sperm count (? raised gonadotrophin secretion) — reverses when treatment ceases.

Drug interactions

Cimetidine inhibits cytochrome P_{450} microsomal enzymes and thus raises blood levels of theophylline, propranolol, phenytoin, warfarin and benzodiazepines.

OTHER H_2 ANTAGONISTS

Ranitidine, famotidine and nizatidine are similar but are not anti-androgenic and do not inhibit drug metabolism.

ANTACIDS

Neutralise HCl and raise gastric pH so reducing irritation and inactivating pepsin but several proteolytic enzymes in gastric juice with activity at high pH. Less effective than cimetidine in suppression of nocturnal acid secretion but similar effect on daytime secretion.

Mainly for symptomatic treatment but given frequently in large doses (enough to neutralise 200 mmol H^+/day) may heal ulcers. Usual doses: between meals and at bedtime but may be taken at hourly or more frequent intervals. GI bleeding associated with severe acute illness may be prevented by antacids.

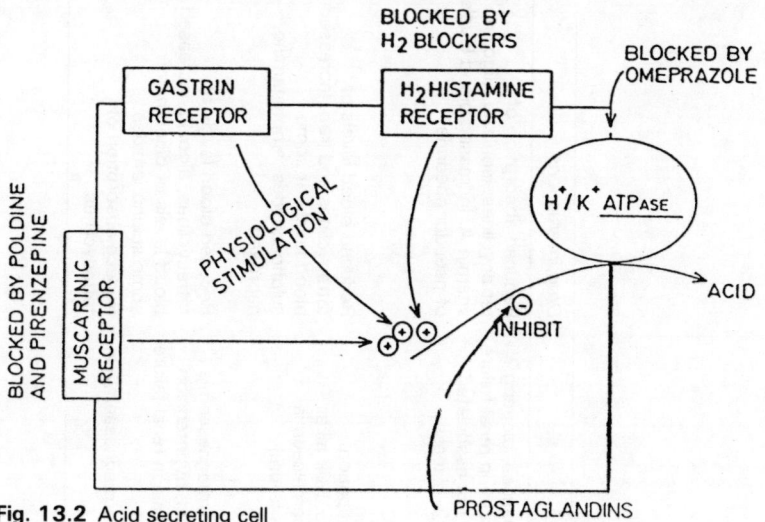

Fig. 13.2 Acid secreting cell

PROTON PUMP INHIBITOR

Omeprazole
Powerful and prolonged block of acid secretion. Omeprazole is the
most effective drug in reflux oesophagitis, in Zollinger–Ellison
syndrome for resistant and recurrent peptic ulcers (particularly if
NSAID are being given). Generally well tolerated. Nausea and
headache are rare.

LIQUORICE DERIVATIVES

Carbenoxolone
Synthetic triterpenoid derived from liquorice root has a steroid-like
molecule. Increases gastric epithelial life span and increases mucus
secretion. Sodium and water retention limits its use. Potassium loss is
stimulated.

Deglycyrrhizinated liquorice
Residue after extraction of glycyrrhizinic acid (precursor of
carbenoxolone) contains substances with less ulcer healing efficacy
than carbenoxolone but which lack its mineralcorticoid action.

BISMUTH CHELATE

Bismuth compounds are weak antacids. Tripotassium dicitrato
bismuthate an alkaline colloidal solution (De-Nol) has been shown to

Table 26 Antacids in common use

Drug	Pharmacology	Adverse effects	Drug interactions
Aluminium hydroxide	Inhibits smooth muscle contraction so delays gastric emptying, decreases gut mobility. Binds bile acids, pepsin, phosphate — latter used to reduce hyperphosphataemia in renal disease	Constipation, nausea, bloating ? Aluminium toxicity in renal failure Administration not associated with Alzheimer's disease	Reduced absorption of tetracyclines, isoniazid, digoxin, vitamin A. Increased blood levels of pseudoephedrine
Calcium carbonate	Produces CO_2 on reaction with HCl. Acid rebound secretion occurs due to local gastrin release + systemic hypercalcaemia. Approx. 40% Ca^{++} absorbed	Belching. Constipation. Hypercalcaemia. Milk-alkali syndrome (hypercalcaemia, calcinosis renal failure)	Reduced blood levels of tatracyclines and iron. Increased blood levels of some sulphonamides, amphetamine, naproxen
Magnesium hydroxide	Most potent H^+ neutralising effect/g of all nonsystemic antacids. Acid rebound is minimal. Stimulates gut mobility.	Diarrhoea, hypermagnesaemia (CNS depression, hypotension, muscle weakness) in renal failure	Reduced blood levels of tetracyclines, digoxin. Increased blood levels of dicoumarol, some sulphonamides
Magnesium trisilicate	Slowly reacts with HCl. Stimulates gut mobility	Diarrhoea, hypermagnesaemia in renal failure	Reduce absorption of tetracyclines

heal D.U. Raises concentrations of mucosal protaglandins and lowers output of pepsin. Also inhibits *Helicobacter pylori*.

No serious acute adverse effects — can turn stools black (confusion with melaena!) and has rather unpleasant taste. Chronic treatment can cause encephalopathy, especially in renal failure. Healing of ulcers is promoted. The relapse rate may be lower than with H_2 blockers.

ANTICHOLINERGIC DRUGS

Reduce gastric acid secretion ('medical vagotomy') and motility and possibly spasm ('antispasmodics').
Non-selective, e.g. poldine; propantheline. Cause dry mouth and skin, thirst, glaucoma, confusion and excitement.

Selective
Pirenzepine is a specific M1 receptor antagonist, ie. it reduces acid secretion without anticholinergic effects on CVS, CNS, eye, gut or bladder.

Causes similar rate of healing of peptic ulcers to H_2 blockers (ie. 60–95% in 8 weeks).

PROSTAGLANDINS

A synthetic analogue of PGE, misoprostol is cytoprotective in the stomach and reduces acid secretion. Can promote healing of duodenal and gastric ulcers and prevent NSAID-induced gastritis and ulceration. Diarrhoea is main toxic effect. It is contraindicated in pregnancy.

SUCRALFATE

Basic aluminium salt of sucrose octasulphate.

Forms chemical complex with protein in ulcer crater by electrostatic interaction to form a protective antacid barrier in ulcer so blocking diffusion of acid and pepsin. Directly inhibits action of pepsin and bile and acts as local antacid (i.e. overall stomach pH unchanged). Also increases gastric mucus and prostaglandins. Sucralfate promotes healing of peptic ulcers at a similar rate to H_2 blockers.

Can very rarely cause aluminium toxicity and gastric bezoar formation. Inhibits the absorption of ciprofloxacin and related drugs.

ANTIBACTERIALS

Bismuth with metronidazole and amoxycillin may prevent recurrence of peptic ulcer disease by destroying *Helicobacter pylori*. Past infections with *H. pylori* are also associated with an increased risk of gastric carcinoma, although the organism is found in 30–70% of adults.

PURGATIVES (LAXATIVES; CATHARTICS)

Avoid unless:
1. straining at stool will cause damage, e.g. postoperatively, in haemorrhoids, post-myocardial infarction
2. in hepatocellular failure
3. occasionally in drug-induced constipation.
   Divided into:
   a. bulk
   b. osmotic
   c. stimulant
   d. lubricant
but some may have more than one type of activity.

Diagnosis of the cause of constipation is important: faecal impaction, obstruction and carcinoma must be excluded. Constipation best treated by increasing fibre and fluid content of diet. Purgatives should be used in lowest dose possible and only for the shortest periods.

BULK PURGATIVES

Contain non-digestible, unabsorbed polysaccharides.

Wheat bran contains 30% fibre. This consists of: cellulose, hemicelluloses, pectins, lignins. These take up water and so increase the bulk of stools. Stretching the colonic wall stimulates peristalsis, thus reducing transit time. Wheat fibre binds bile salts and increases their excretion. However, blood cholesterol is not reduced on a bran-supplemented diet, although this does occur with guar gum or fruit pectin.

Bran either native or as tablets is given in divided doses 12–24 g/day with fluid. Acts within 24–72 hours.

Bran is of value in treating:
> constipation
> diverticulosis
> spastic colon
> ulcerative colitis.

It probably could play a role in preventing:
> haemorrhoids
> anal fissure
> appendicitis
> diverticulitis.

It has been suggested that it may reduce the likelihood of:
> varicose veins
> cholecystitis
> carcinoma of the colon
> coronary artery disease
> obesity.

Table 27 Purgatives

Drug	Pharmacological properties	Approximate dose effect interval	Toxicity	Special uses
OSMOTIC PURGATIVES				
Sodium sulphate	Increased bulk of water in lumen stimulates peristalsis	2 h	Sodium absorption	
Magnesium sulphate	Like sodium sulphate, in addition Mg stimulates peristalsis by liberating cholecystokinin	2 h	Magnesium can be absorbed and be of clinical significance in renal failure	Hepatocellular failure
Lactulose	Dissacharide split by bacteria in colon to organic acids which are unabsorbed and act osmotically to increase bulk of stools. Gas formation is increased	46 h	Contraindicated in galactosaemia	Hepatocellular failure
CHEMICAL STIMULANTS OF COLON				
Senna	Contains glycosides which are hydrolysed by colonic bacteria to sennosides A and B. These are absorbed and then stimulate colonic peristalsis by acting on mural nerve plexuses. Enters milk	8 h	Griping and diarrhoea. Diarrhoea in suckling child. Melanosis coli. Red or yellow coloration of urine	
Bisacodyl	Deacetylated in gut, absorbed, glucuronidated in liver and enters enterohepatic circulation. Has a direct action on gut wall and reaches gut wall in arterial blood	10 h	Abdominal cramps	Can be given by suppository

Table 27 (continued)

Drug	Pharmacological properties	Approximate dose effect interval	Toxicity	Special uses
Phenolphthalein	15% absorbed from gut, excreted in bile and undergoes an enterohepatic circulation — resulting in a prolonged effect. Active fraction produced in liver and undergoes further modification in colon	8–10 h	4% develop a fixed drug eruption. Other rashes. SLE-like syndrome. Alkaline urine coloured pink	Not recommended.
LUBRICANTS AND STOOL SOFTENERS				
Dioctyl sodium sulphosuccinate (DSS: dioctyl)	Surface agent allows water into inspissated colonic contents	1 day	Detergent action alters intestinal mucosa permeability	Faecal impaction
Liquid paraffin	Lubricates contents of colon. Not digested	1 day	Interferes with absorption of fat soluble vitamins. Aspiration lipid pneumonia. Anal leakage. Absorption into tissues (e.g. after intestinal operations). Can cause granuloma formation. Possible carcinogenicity	(Should not be used)

Adverse effects
Flatulence
Reduced absorption of calcium and iron
Avoid in coeliac disease and gluten enteropathy
If taken with insufficient fluid may form masses in gut and produce obstruction.
Other bulk purgatives with similar effects (used if bran not tolerated) are ispaghula husk, methylcellulose and sterculia.

Table 28 Symptomatic drug treatment of diarrhoea

Drug	Dose	Special features	Adverse effects	Mechanism of action
Codeine phosphate	45–120 mg daily in 4–8-hourly doses	Tolerance and dependence can occur rarely. Contraindicated in hepatic or diverticular disease	Nausea, dizziness and sedation. Constipation	Opiates decrease propulsive and increase tonic gut contractions allowing prolonged contact of mucosa and greater water absorption
Diphenoxylate HCl	10 mg start then 5 mg 6-hourly	Pethidine derivative — dependance can occur. Contraindicated by hepatic or diverticular disease. Also with small doses of atropine as Lomotil and Reasec — dangerous in overdose especially in children	Euphoria, nausea, dizziness and sedation. Rarely ileus	As codeine
Loperamide HCl	4 mg start then 2 mg after each loose stool up to total 16 daily	No CNS effects — so no synergism with tranquillizers, sedatives or alcohol. No major anticholinergic actions	Occasionally dry-mouth, headache, dizziness, vomiting, abdominal colic	Interacts with cholinergic and non-cholinergic mechanisms in gut wall to inhibit motility
Cholestyramine	12–24 g daily 4–8 hourly	Used only for diarrhoea after ileal resection, vagotomy, bile acid malabsorption	See hypercholesterolaemia	Basic anion-exchange resin to bind bile salts preventing reabsorpton. So used for bile acid diarrhoea

TREATMENT OF ACUTE DIARRHOEAL SYNDROMES

Replace lost fluid and electrolytes
Most attacks are self-limiting.
   Consider use of symptomatic treatment with codeine,
diphenoxylate etc, or with an absorbent mixture such as:
1. kaolin
2. chalk
3. methylcelluose — useful in control of ileostomy and colostomy
4. sterculia — useful in control ileostomy and colostomy.
Chemotherapy is indicated for:
1. *Shigellosis* — only severe, invasive cases with systemic
   manifestations require chemotherapy: ampicillin 2–4 g/day;
   cotrimoxazole tablets 2, 12-hourly.
2. *Enteric fever* — chloramphenicol, ciprofloxacin, amoxycillin or
   ampicillin.
3. *Salmonella food poisoning* — only when septicaemia occurs then
   amoxycillin, ampicillin, trimethoprim or ciprofloxacin used.
4. *Cholera* — toxin increases adenyl cyclase activity raising cyclic
   AMP which reduces Na^+ absorption and increases Cl^- and HCO_3
   secretion by gut. Na^+ absorption encouraged by giving oral
   glucose/saline: glucose and Na^+ absorption are coupled together
   in mucosal cells. Give mixture of 4 g NaCl, 4 g $NaHCO_3$, 1 g KCl,
   20 g glucose in 1 litre water — may need 10–15 litres in 24 hours.
   Oral teracycline eliminates vibrio and reduces toxin formation but
   tetracycline resistant strains have appeared in Bangladesh.
5. *Campylobacter enteritis* can be treated with erythromycin or
   ciprofloxacin.

Traveller's diarrhoea
Various causes: toxigenic *E. coli*, Shigella, *Giardia lamblia*, Salmonella,
Entamoeba histolytica, Campylobacter jejuni, Vibrio spp., rotavirus,
Norwalk agent and *Cryptosporidium spp.*
   Acute onset of watery diarrhoea and abdominal cramps occurring a
few days after arrival, usually self-limiting. Doxycycline,
cotrimoxazole; trimethoprim, norfloxacin and mecillinam may protect
but many organisms are resistant and drug toxicity and drug
resistance can be caused. Bismuth subsalicylate is also of value in
prophylaxis.

Treatment
Replace fluid and electrolytes orally.
Avoid drugs inhibiting intestinal mobility which prevents elimination of
pathogens, causes gut stasis and may extend the period of illness.
Post-infective malabsorption can be precipitated by some
antiperistaltic agents.

SULPHASALAZINE

70% reaches colon and then is split by bacteria to 5-aminosalicylate and sulphapyridine.

Acts by inhibiting prostaglandin synthase and 5-lipoxygenase. This inhibits synthesis of prostaglandins and leukotrienes. Also blocks the formation of chemoattractants for neutrophils. Acts as a scavenger for oxygen-free radicals.

Uses
Ulcerative colitis — reduces frequency and severity of recurrences
Crohn's disease of colon — used in acute attacks
Rheumatoid arthritis
Radiation enteritis

Adverse effects
Allergy to sulphanamide component.
Dose-dependent effects: nausea, vomiting, headaches, fever, arthralgia, transient leucocytosis, bluish colour of skin, reversible male sterility, haemolytic anaemia in G6PD deficiency, pericarditis, pancreatitis, pleurisy.

Mesalazine and olsalazine
Deliver 5-aminosalicylic acid to the colon without the unwanted effects of sulphapyridine. Used for patients intolerant to sulphasalazine and men who want to be fertile.

Treatment of ulcerative colitis
Avoid salicylates as these can aggravate diarrhoea.
A. *Mild attacks* without systemic features, usually confined to rectum and sigmoid colon. Can often be managed as out-patients.
1. Sulphasalazine usually oral. Topical (enema) also effective in distal disease.
2. Topical corticosteroid — Prednisolone disodium phosphate suppositories 2, once or twice daily or as enema.
3. If 1 and 2 ineffective, prednisolone 40 mg/day p.o.

B. *Moderately severe attacks* — some systemic upset usually involving at least the left side and sigmoid colon and rectum and requiring hospital admission.
1. Prednisolone 40 mg/day p.o
2. Replacement of fluid, electrolytes, iron and blood as required. Possibly parenteral feeding.
3. If no response, intravenous hydrocortisone or oral prednisolone.

As patient improves prednisolone dose slowly reduced, topical corticosteroids and sulphasalazine begun. Up to 20% of topical hydrocortisone is absorbed. Beclomethasone and budenoside are more potent topical agents with less systemic absorption (high first pass metabolism).

C. *Severe attacks* with major systemic effects and bowel involvement.
1. Prednisolone-21-phosphate 60 mg i.v./day, hydrocortisone hemisuccinate 300–400 mg i.v./day or oral prednisolone.
2. Replacement of fluid, electrolytes and blood.
3. Parenteral feeding.
4. Collaborative management with surgeons.

D. *Maintenance of remission.*
1. Sulphasalazine is the only drug clearly shown as effective prophylactic but it is ineffective in significant relapse: the converse applies to steroids. Mesalazine and olsalazine are alternatives.
2. Azathioprine or mercaptopurine may be steroid spacing in refractory disease. Low dose methotrexate or cyclosporin may produce improvement in severe colitis.
3. Avoid precipitating factors: intestinal infections, stress, 20% have milk intolerance.
4. Prompt treatment of impending relapse.

E. *Systemic manifestations*
Arthritis; sacroilitis; ankylosing spondylitis; erythema nodosum; pyoderma gangrenosum; iritis; urethritis; chronic active hepatitis.
   These are all indications for coticosteroid treatment.

Treatment of Crohn's disease
A. *Acute attack*
1. Bed rest.
2. Codeine phosphate or diphenoxylate.
3. If severe or no response, prednisolone 40–60 mg oral. Mainly effective in small bowel disease.
4. Sulphasalazine may improve acute attacks of colonic Crohn's disease.

B *Prevention of relapse and treatment in remission*
1. Sulphasalazine much less effective than in ulcerative colitis.
2. Azathioprine, mercaptopurine, cyclosporin and methotrexate have been used but carry greater hazard.
3. Metronidazole for symptomatic perianal and colonic disease.
4. Diarrhoea may result from fat malabsorption and may respond to a low fat or medium chain triglyceride diet. Alternatively it may result from bile salt colitis due to terminal ileitis or a blind loop syndrome: these may respond to cholestyramine.
   Otherwise symptomatic treatment with codeine phosphate, Lomotil or methylcellulose.
5. Pain, if not due to obstruction, is treated with a mild analgesic;

sometimes mebeverine helps. Exclusion of milk or an elemental diet may help.

Treatment of irritable bowel syndrome.

1. Dietary
   — high fibre diets using bran (12–24 g/day)
   — reduced sugar diets
   — eliminate lactose in lactase-deficient patients.
2. Simple psychotherapy.
3. Anticholinergic drugs if above fail. No evidence that any is better than atropine but commonly used are propantheline, mepenzolate and dicyclomine.
4. Smooth muscle relaxants without anticholinergic properties may relieve pain. Mebeverine and enteric coated peppermint oil are both effective.
5. Psychotropic agents, e.g. amitriptyline, imipramine which also have anticholinergic activity have been used as adjunctive treatments.

HEPATIC ENCEPHALOPATHY

A. Precipitating factors of encephalopathy (in approximate order of frequency) in patients with chronic liver disease

Factor	Presumed mechanism
Uraemia	Ureases in gut split area to NH_3
Sedatives, analgesics	Direct CNS depression. Impaired hepatic drug metabolism
GI haemorrhage	Blood is substrate for NH_3 production in gut. Shock, hypoxia and hypovolaemia impair CNS and hepatic function
Hypokalaemia/diuretics	Hypokalaemia and alkalosis decrease renal NH_3 loss. Alkalosis increases NH_3 entry into CNS. Vigorous diuresis produces hypovolaemia and impaired cardiac, CNS, hepatic and renal function
Excess dietary protein	Substrate for NH_3 production — especially in patients with porto-caval shunt
Infection	Tissue catabolism increases NH_3 Dehydration, hypotension, hypoxia

NB Drugs to be avoided or given in reduced dose in patients with liver disease:
1. Opioids.
2. Sedatives and neuroleptics.
3. Ethanol: acute alcoholism precipitates encephalopathy by reducing hepatic and cerebral function.

4. Diuretics: Thiazides and loop diuretics (but amiloride and spironolactone can be used with care).

B. Treatment of acute hepatic failure and encephalopathy (in ICU)
1. Remove or treat precipitating causes. Treat cerebral oedema with dexamethasone.
2. Reduce NH_3 production.
   a. No protein. High carbohydrate diet prevents protein catabolism and NH_3 production — 1500 ml fluid, 1000 cals, 200 g carbohydrate in 24 hours given i.v. or p.o.
   b. $MgSO_4$ purge.
   c. Empty colon with enemas.
   d. Alter colonic flora and reduce toxin absorption: give lactulose and neomycin orally.
3. Correct metabolic/respiratory disturbances
   a. Electrolytes:
      hyponatraemia (partly dilutional, partly shift into cells)
      hypokalaemia
   b. Acid-base disturbances — respiratory and metabolic alkalosis early, metabolic acidosis late.
   c. Hypoxia — give oxygen by mask or intermittent positive-pressure ventilation with PEEP.
   d. Hypoglycaemia can develop rapidly. Treat with intravenous glucose.
   e. Watch for acute tubular necrosis or pre-renal failure.
4. Control haematological disturbances. Give H_2 blocker for gastrointestinal haemorrhage.
5. Be wary of infection, cardiac arrhythmias, cerebral oedema and pulmonary oedema.

C. Treatment of chronic hepatic failure and encephalopathy
1. Avoid precipitating factors, eg. alcohol.
2. Diet: re-introduce protein (vegetable rather than animal) 20 g alternate days to limit of tolerance (usually 20–40 g/day).
3. Oral lactulose.
4. If evidence of infection (e.g. unexplained hypotension) then i.v. antibacterials.
5. Ascites: no diuretics till encephalopathy cleared. Can remove up to 2 litres to help breathing.
6. Defective haemostasis: fresh frozen plasma; vitamin K, calcium gluconate.

D. Treatment of cirrhotic oedema and ascites
1. General:
   a. Bed rest with daily measurement of weight, girth, electrolytes and fluid balance

   b. Salt restriction (no added salt = 50 mmol/day; low salt
      diet = 20 mmol/day)
   c. Fluid restriction < 1500 ml/day
2. Diuretics:
   — if trial of general measures fails
   — avoid weight loss > 1.5 kg/day
   — avoid hypokalaemia and hyperkalaemia
   — remember ascites may not need aggressive treatment, that
   diuretics can cause complications and do not increase life
   expectancy.
   a. Spironolactone (begin with 100–200 mg/day but can increase
      slowly)
   b. If these fail add frusemide (up to 120 mg/day) cautiously.
3. Infuse salt-free albumin if hypoalbuminaemia a major factor but
   effect usually transient.
4. Paracentesis for symptomatic relief. Total paracentesis with
   albumin infusion.
5. Ascites ultrafiltration and re-infusion.
6. Non-selective (total) shunts; selective (distal spleno-renal) shunts;
   devascularisation (oesophageal transection).

E. Management of bleeding oesophageal varices
1. Admit to hospital. Managed by a joint medical-surgical team. Initial
   clinical, haematological and biochemical assessment.
2. Correct hypovolaemia, treat suspected sepsis. H_2 blocker only if
   bleeding from a gastric erosion.
3. Control of bleeding in order of preference:
   a. Vasopressin 20 units in 100 ml 5% destrose given i.v. over
      15 mins. Causes intense splanchic vasoconstriction and
      reduces hepatic portal blood flow. Also gives colic, facial pallor,
      and rarely hypertension and angina. Nitroglycerine skin patches
      to reduce systemic vasoconstriction.
   b. Balloon tamponade controls bleeding in 90% of cases.
   c. Surgical and endoscopic procedures.
4. Treatment for acute encephalopathy usually required.
5. Non-specific β-blockade or sclerotherapy may reduce chance of
   rebleeding.

MEDICAL TREATMENT OF GALLSTONES

Cholesterol stones comprise 75% of all gall stones: these alone are
amenable to dissolution by medical treatment. Result from secretion
of cholesterol-saturated bile by the liver but cause of this
super-saturation is uncertain. Cholesterol stones may be dissolved by
making bile unsaturated with respect to cholesterol so that cholesterol
in the stones redissolves in bile acid and phospholipid micelles.
   Medical treatment offered if there are no acute symptoms, there is
a functioning gallbladder and the patient is unfit or refuses surgery.

CHENODEOXYCHOLIC ACID

Reduces biliary cholesterol saturation by reducing hepatic cholesterol synthesis — inhibits hydroxymethylglutaryl coenzyme-A reductase (HMGCoAR), the rate-limiting enzyme for cholesterol synthesis from acetate. May act directly or via its metabolite ursodeoxycholic acid. Also increases the bile acid pool.

Well absorbed orally, undergoes enterohepatic circulation. In successful treatments stones disappear in 2 years. Ineffective in pigment stones, calcified stones and stones with a diameter over 1.5 cm. Stones frequently recur within a few years.

Adverse effects
1. Diarrhoea (about 30–40%).
2. Transiently raised serum transaminase levels without evidence of liver damage.

URSODEOXYCHOLIC ACID

Similar mode of action to chenodeoxycholic acid of which it is a metabolite. May be more active inhibitor of HMGCoAR.

Patients selected as for chenodeoxycholic acid.

ROWACHOL

Proprietary mixture of terpenes which is less effective than the above two drugs. May be used as additional treatment.

Methyl-tert-butyl ether (MTBE)
Is a dissolver of gall stones when introduced into the gall bladder endoscopically or via percutaneous catheterisation.

14. Obesity, vitamins, hyperlipoproteinaemias and nutrition

TREATMENT OF OBESITY

1. Dieting
a. Assess calorie needs and what patient consumes.
b. Put on a *balanced* diet with a deficit of 500 cal/day (should lose 0.5 kg/week). Total starvation not recommended because long term success is low and risks are high; unbalanced diets (e.g. grapefruits only; low carbohydrate) lead to nutritional and intestinal problems. To lose a kg needs an energy deficit of 700 kcals.
c. Teach patient to count calories; particular care to include sweet drinks; alcohol; sugar in tea and coffee; fat used in cooking.
d. Change patterns of eating:
   Antecedent events (e.g. attractive adverts, visits to food shops) must be recognised.
   Behaviour of eating — learn only to eat at mealtimes and sitting at a table. No standing in kitchen or by 'fridge. Have breakfast but no snack after evening meal. Making a complete list of what is eaten can alone improve eating pattern. Also keeping a record of hunger helps to space meals.
   Consequences of eating — understanding the depressive effect of guilt about breaking diet. Rewards include improved appearance and interpersonal relationships.

2. Exercise
Not only increases calorie consumption, but may readjust appetite to match energy needs. Strenuous physical exercise hazardous for grossly obese, but a planned progressive programme used. 'Aerobic' exercise *daily* for at least 45 mins.

3. Drugs
Controversial (but patients lose 0.25 kg/week more than those receiving placebo).
a. Thyroid hormones — only large doses are effective and produce no dependence. However, lean bodyweight also

decreased and cardiac toxicity likely. Not recommended.
   b. Diethylpropion, phentermine, mazindol: effective but produce
      excitement, tolerance, risk of dependence. Cannot be used
      with MAOI, in CVS disorder (including hypertension). They are
      seldom indicated, and should only be used under close
      specialist supervision.
   c. Fenfluramine, a 5HT agonist, is anorectic but sedative. Can
      precipitate depression. Dexfenfluramine is the active isomer of
      fenfluramine. It is said to have less adverse effects than the
      racemic mixture.
   d. Bulk agents (cellulose, guar gum, sterculia, bran) not shown to
      be effecitve.

4. Surgery
   a. Intestinal bypass: lose 5–70 kg in first year.
      Disadvantages: haemorrhoids; fluid and electrolyte imbalance;
      protein malnutrition; liver failure; renal stones; metabolic bone
      disease; polyarthritis. Mortality is 3%.
   b. Vertical band gastroplasty.
   c. Jaw wiring: lose 20 kg in first 5 months.
      Disadvantages: dental damage; risk of aspiration; gain weight
      when wires removed.

VITAMINS

Vitamin A
A number of forms of vitamin A exist, e.g.:
   retinol (vitamin A_1)
   3-dehydroretinol (vitamin A_2)
   retinoic acid (vitamin A acid).

Deficiency
1. Earliest signs: follicular hyperkeratosis and infections of skin.
2. Reduced visual dark adaptation is a feature of severe lack.
   Permanent blindness follows prolonged deficiency.
3. Blindness may also be the result of keratomalacia, xerophthalmia
   and corneal scarring.
4. Bronchorespiratory keratinisation, mucus plugging and infections.
5. Urinary calculi; impaired spermatogenesis.
6. Metaplasia of pancreatic duct epithelium; diarrhoea.
7. Skin: atrophy of sweat glands; papular rashes.
8. Bone: increased formation of cancellous bone.
9. Sense organs: decreased hearing, taste, smell, + 2 and 3.

Hypervitaminosis
Usually due to excess intake of retinol with a relative lack of vitamin E.

Chronic:
1. Irritability; headache, fatigue.
2. Anorexia, vomiting.
3. Dry itching skin, skin desquamation, erythema.
4. Loss of body hair, deposition of carotenoids.
5. Myalgia, pain in feet and legs.
6. Gingivitis, mouth fissures.
7. Nystagmus, papilloedema.
8. Enlargement of liver, spleen and lymph nodes.
Acute:
1. Drowsiness.
2. Headache, vomiting, papilloedema (bulging fontanelle in infants).
3. Desquamation of skin.
Uses:
1. Prevention of deficiency: normal daily requirement 800 r.e. for women; 100 r.e. for men (r.e. = 1 retinol equivalent = 1 μg retinol = 1 unit of vitamin A).
2. In severe deficiency (e.g. Kwashiorkor): a single i.m. injection of 30 mg retinol (as palmitate), then 60–120 mg retinol every 3–6 months. Reduces the mortality of measles in deficient children.
3. Desquamation of skin, e.g. in Darier's disease; ichthyoses and severe psoriasis: retinoic acid (tretinoin) or etretinate (Tigason) for 2–4 weeks. Oral isotretinoin (13-cis-retinoic acid) for severe cystic acne.
4. Topical tretinoin for acne vulgaris.

Ascorbic acid (vitamin C)

Ascorbic acid deficiency
Dietary lack in elderly, alcoholics, drug addicts, infants on poor diets.
1. Perifollicular hyperkeratosis in skin.
2. Petechiae and ecchymoses in skin.
3. Slowed healing of wounds.
4. Loose teeth, gingivitis, bleeding gums.
5. Anaemia.
6. In babies: irritability, painful sub-periosteal haemorrhages.

Toxicity
Excessive doses may produce dysuria, oxalate kidney stones and interfere with anticoagulant action — but such toxic effects are uncommon.

Uses
1. Prevention of scurvy: 60 mg ascorbic acid daily (increased needs: smokers, oral contraceptive use, infections, wound healing). Usual route is oral.

2. Malabsorption and during parenteral nutrition i.m. or i.v. 200 mg sodium ascorbate/day.
3. Idiopathic methaemoglobinaemia: 150 mg ascorbic acid/day.
4. Prevention and/or cure respiratory viral infections: large dose used — results are inconclusive (high doses in pregnancy can produce rebound scurvy in offspring).

HYPERLIPOPROTEINAEMIAS (HYPERLIPIDAEMIAS)

Steps in management
1. Confirm raised blood lipid(s) and look for treatable underlying cause (diabetes, alcohol, hypothyroidism).
2. Family history and investigation for raised lipids, early CVS disease and pancreatitis. Rule out secondary hypercholesterolaemia (hypothyroidism, diabetes).
3. Treat to prevent atherosclerosis and pancreatitis (LDL cholesterol and triglycerides respectively).
4. If decide to treat try diet first.
5. If 4 fails try 4 plus drugs.
6. Look out for and treat other modifiable risk factors for atheroma (hypertension, smoking).

Decide to treat:
1. Young patients with hypercholesterolaemia or hypertriglyceridaemia with family history of early atheromatous disease.
2. All patients with serum triglycerides above 15–20 mmol/l.
3. Intensity of treatment depends on the plasma cholesterol concentration and on the coexistence of other cardiovascular risk factors. In borderline cases the decision whether to use drugs is helped by knowing the HDL as well as LDL cholesterol.

Diet
1. Primary lipoprotein lipase deficiency: very low fat diet.
2. All other types:
   a. treat obesity with calorie restriction and exercise
   b. reduce dietary saturated fats. Total fats restricted to 30% of calorie intake
   c. partially replace b. with unsaturated fats
   d. increase complex (starchy) carbohydrate content of diet to 55–60% of total calories. Include pectins and other gel forming fibres.
   e. vegetable proteins to replace animal proteins
   f. restrict sugar and alcohol.

Drugs
1. **Cholestyramine** and **colestipol** are resins which bind to bile salts in the intestine. They can cause abdominal distension, constipation

and rarely steatorrhoea. They induce a modest fall in serum cholesterol and reduce the risk of myocardial infarction. They may raise serum triglycerides.

2. **Fibrates** (gemfibrozil, bezafibrate) also cause a modest reduction in serum cholesterol, and gemfibrozil has been shown to reduce the risk of myocardial infarction. They cause a much greater fall in triglyceride concentration and are particularly useful with severe hypertriglyceridaemia (when this is not due to alcohol consumption).

3. **HMGCoA reductase inhibitors** (simvastatin, pravastatin) cause a greater fall in serum cholesterol (approximately 30% drop in LDL-cholesterol). They have yet to be proved effective in reducing the risk of myocardial infarction. They cause increased hepatic LDL uptake as a result of increased expression of LDL receptors on hepatocyte surface membranes. Consequently they are not effective in homozygous familial hypercholesterolaemia in which LDL receptors are absent. They are synergistic with bile acid binding resins.

4. **Nicotinic acid.** Lowers both cholesterol and triglycerides. Useful in resistant familial hypercholesterolaemia (with resins) and in combined hyperlipidaemia (with resins if necessary). Toxicity includes flushing, dyspepsia, palpitations, itching and aggravation of diabetes. Flushing is prostaglandin mediated and can be blocked with aspirin.

5. **Fish oil concentrates** rich in eicosapentaenoic acid reduce serum triglycerides but not cholesterol. These may be used in patients with hypertriglyceridaemia and recurrent pancreatitis. It is also possible that fish oil may reduce the risk of cardiovascular disease as a result of effects on thromboxane and prostacyclin biosynthesis.

ENTERAL NUTRITION

Used to provide calories and nitrogen if a negative balance has occurred due to starvation, trauma, infection, burns or surgery. Also used in malabsorption, post-gastrectomy and dysphagia. Cheaper and safer than parenteral nutrition.

Usual daily adult need: 8–20 g nitrogen in 1500–4000 cals (6270–16720 kJ). Administration best via small (1 mm) bore tube with continuous gravity feed.

Toxicity

Lactose intolerance (Asians and Africans esp). can cause diarrhoea — if likely choose lactose-free solution.

Abdominal distension, colic, diarrhoea (usually when full strength feeds introduced too rapidly).

Tube problems (e.g. irritation, ulceration of oesophagus, accidental insertion into lung).

Some proprietary enteral feeds

Name	Energy content	Additional features
Clinifeed 400	1674 kJ/375 ml tin 593 kJ/gN = 142 cals/gN	Complete nutrition Casein is protein source Gluten free
Ensure	450 kJ/100 ml 643 kJ/gN = 154 cals/gN	Complete nutrition Casein and soya protein Gluten and lactose free
Flexical	1850 kJ/100 ml 1070 kJ/gN = 256 cals/gN	Complete nutrition Casein amino acids Gluten and lactose free
Forceval	1540 kJ/100 g	Low fat. Gluten and lactose free
Isocal	445 kJ/100 ml	Complete nutrition Casein and soya protein Gluten and lactose free

Hyperglycaemia (give insulin to keep blood glucose normal).
Low blood levels of K, Ca, Mg, Zn, PO_4 (measure these × 2 weekly)
Abnormal liver function tests.

Chronic renal failure and hepatic failure
Require high energy, low fluid and low electrolyte diet, e.g.:
Caloreen (polyglucose polymer, low in electrolytes, low protein,
lactose and fructose free) 1.67 mJ/100 g.
Hycal (carbohydrate as corn syrup, lactose, fructose, sucrose, protein
free. Low in electrolytes) 1.03 mJ/100 ml.

PARENTERAL NUTRITION
Only used when the enteral route cannot be used in malnourished
patients.

Requirements

1. Nitrogen
As crystalline L-amino acid mixtures (not partial hydrolysates of whole
protein).
   Essential amino acids should be approx. 40% (w/w) of total. Higher
proportion of branched amino acids (valine, leucine, and isoleucine)
lower proportion of phenylalanine and tyrosine in liver failure, sepsis
and severe injuries. Several formulations are available, including:

Synthamin 9 (9.3 gN/l)   also contain Na, K, Cl, Mg, PO_4,
Synthamin 14 (14.4 gN/l)   acetate (but also electrolyte free)
Synthamin 17 (17.9 gN/l)
Vamin N (9.4 gN/l also contains Na, K, Cl, Mg, Ca (with or without
                      glucose and fructose)

2. Energy
As glucose *or* glucose plus lipid. Basal requirement is 25 cal/kg/day
and the usual need is 150–250 cals (627–1045 kJ) of non-protein
energy/k nitrogen supplied.

In severely negative nitrogen balance, only glucose is used, but in
other types of patient the combination is given because less water
retention results. i.v. lipid preparations:
Intralipid 10% (soya bean oil + egg phospholipid) emulsion 4620 kJ/l
Intralipid 20% (soya been oil + egg phospholipid) emulsion 8400 kJ/l.

3. Vitamins
Recommended daily intake:

retinol	700 IU
thiamine	1.4 mg
riboflavin	2.1 mg
nicotinamide	14 mg
pyridoxine	2.1 mg
folic acid	2 mg
cyanocobalamin	2.0 μg
biotin	350 μg
pantothenic acid	14 mg
ascorbic acid	35 mg
calciferol	100 IU
tocopheryl acetate	30 IU
phytomenaquinone	140 μg

Preparations include:
Multibionta   none are ideal, e.g. take care not to give
Parentrovite   excess retinol. Supplements of
Solvito   vitamins and ascorbic acid for
                         alcoholic and catabolic patients.

PANCREATIC ENZYME REPLACEMENT

Used in pancreatic insufficiency due to cystic fibrosis, chronic
pancreatitis etc to reduce diarrhoea, steatorrhoea and weight loss.
Pancreatin B.P. contains proteases, lipases and amylase — available
as enteric and sugar-coated (e.g. Pancrex V) capsules, enteric-coated

granules to be taken dry or with liquid (e.g. Protopan) or capsules to be opened and spinkled on food (e.g. Cotazym). Usual dose is 2–8 g in divided dose. Concurrent use of cimetidine to reduce gastric acidity improves delivery of intact enzyme to the duodenum. Adverse effects include irritation of skin surrounding mouth and anus; hyperuricosuria and uric acid stones (in children with cystic fibrosis ingesting excessive amounts of purine-containing pancreatic extract).

Patients also require supplemental water and fat-soluble vitamins.

15. Drugs affecting the blood

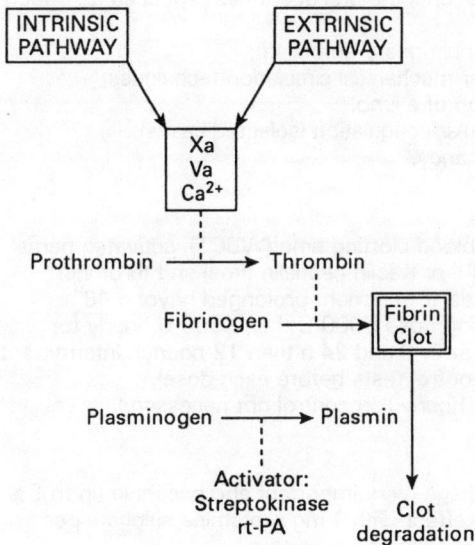

Fig. 15.1 Coagulation pathways.

COAGULATION PATHWAYS

ANTICOAGULANTS

Drugs affecting the clotting process.

1. Heparin
A mixture of sulphated polysaccharides (MV 6000–20 000)
120 U = 1 mg. Active in vitro and in vivo. Acts immediately.

Action
Heparin greatly accelerates the action of antithrombin III. It is therefore ineffective in individuals with antithrombin III deficiency.

Pharmacokinetics
Precipitated by gastric acid, but can be absorbed from s.c., i.m. or i.v. injection (but i.m. commonly causes haematomas and so not used) $T\frac{1}{2}$ = 60–90 mins. Does not cross placental barrier or enter milk.

Indications
When oral anticoagulants are used, heparin may be given during the first 36 h of treatment (i.e. until the oral agent has produced its effect) (see warfarin);
　　deep vein thrombosis; pulmonary embolism;
　　haemodialysis and other mechanical circulation techniques;
　　acute arterial obstruction of a limb;
　　disseminated intravascular coagulation (selected cases);
　　anticoagulation in pregnancy.

Dose and control of dose
Heparin prolongs: whole blood clotting time (WBCT), activated partial thromboplastin time (APTT or Kaolin-cephalin time) and thrombin time. Control tests essential if treatment prolonged beyond 48 h. Continuous infusion: loading dose 5000 U then 1500 U hourly for 7–10 days (control tests at 0, 6 and 24 h then 12-hourly). Intermittent i.v.: 10 000 U 6-hourly (control tests before each dose). Low dose s.c.: 5000 U 4 hourly (lab control not necessary).

Toxicity
1. Spontaneous haemorrhage (very important and occurs in up to 5% of patients) — reverse effect with 1 mg protamine sulphate per 100 U heparin given over the previous hour.
2. Allergy (uncommon).
3. Osteoporosis (chronic administration of 10 000 U daily).
4. Alopecia (rare).
5. Thrombocytopenia.

2. Oral anticoagulants (vitamin K antagonists)
Warfarin is almost invariably the first choice. Other oral anticoagulants (e.g. phenindione) are used for patients with idiosyncratic reactions to warfarin.

Actions
Maximum effect 3–5 days after starting treatment. Warfarin inhibits vitamin K epoxide reductase, thereby blocking the conversion of vitamin K epoxide to the reduced form (vitamin KH_2). The reduced

vitamin is the cofactor for carboxylation of glutamate residues in the inactive proenzyme forms of factors II, VII, IX and X, as well as anticoagulant proteins (proteins C and S). Through the post translational modification of these residues, the proteins acquire metal binding properties which result in a conformational change on binding to calcium. This is necessary for them to bind to their cofactors on physiological surfaces.

Pharmacokinetics
Complete absorption from gut. All oral anticoagulants enter the fetus. Warfarin is 97% bound to plasma albumin. Warfarin: mean $T\frac{1}{2} = 44$ h (but 12-fold variation). Eliminated by hepatic microsomal metabolism. Phenindiones (but very little warfarin) enter breast milk.
   Warfarin is racemic — S and R form: S isomer 3–4 × more potent but rapidly metabolised. Main metabolite of S isomer is 7-hydroxywarfarin. Main metabolite of R isomer is warfarin alcohol. Phenylbutazone reduces metabolism of S warfarin and increases metabolism of R warfarin — net effect is same amount of racemic warfarin but more anticoagulation (because S more active).

Indications
Much difference of opinion.
Limited administration:
   prophylaxis of thromboembolic disease
   deep vein thrombosis — 2 weeks treatment or longer
   pulmonary embolism — 6 weeks to 6 months treatment
   preparatory to cardioversion

Long term or permanent administration:
   atrial fibrillation or a large left atrium
   artificial heart valves.

Contraindications
Active bleeding, e.g. ulcerative colitis, peptic ulcer, haematuria
Haemorrhagic diathesis
Dissecting aneurysm
Surgery of CNS or eye
Potential bleeding lesion, e.g. papilloma of bladder, history of peptic
   ulcer
Uncontrolled severe hypertension
Diabetes, especially with retinopathy
Alcoholism
Pregnancy
Hepatic or renal insufficiency
Poor patient compliance.

   Increased susceptibility in old age with increased risks of falls and head injury.

Dose and control of dose
Prothrombin time increases with reduced activity of factors II, VII, X. Variations between laboratories have been largely overcome by the adoption of an International Normalised Ratio (INR) system. This involves calibration of the thromboplastin used against a reference preparation. Initial daily dose of warfarin is 10 mg. After 48 h INR used to modify dose. At first daily tests carried out — but when anticoagulation established, every 4–12 weeks. Therapeutic range for most indications is a target INR of 2.0–3.0.

Toxicity
1. Haemorrhage (very important and common: 5% per treatment year). Effect terminated by oral or i.v. vitamin K (5–25 mg) or water soluble analogue (e.g. phytomenadione 10–20 mg; menadiol diphosphate 10–100 mg). Check prothrombin time at 3 h and repeat if very prolonged. Prothrombin time returns to normal in 12–36 h. If a more rapid effect is needed (e.g. with increasing bleeding) then immediate reversal is possible using fresh frozen plasma or clotting factor concentrates.
2. Coumarins: skin and fat necrosis; alopecia; abortion; congenital abnormalities (nasal hypoplasia). Skin necrosis results from thrombosis in venules in subcutaneous tissues in especially, breast, buttock and penis. There is an association with protein C or protein S deficiency although this complication can develop in people without such deficiencies. The effect is rare but devastating.
3. Phenindiones: block I_2 uptake by thyroid; uricosuria; congenital nasal abnormalities; renal tubular damage; hepatitis; dermatitis; agranulocytosis; pink urine (fades with acetic acid); up to 3% of patients on phenindione develop sensitivity reactions.

Oral anticoagulants — interactions
1. Pharmacokinetic

a. *Enhanced effect*
Stereoselective inhibition of metabolism of active (S) isomer: metronidazole, phenylbutazone, co-trimoxazole.

Stereoselective inhibition of metabolism of inactive (R) isomer (little effect): cimetidine, omeprazole.

Non-stereoselective inhibition of metabolism: amiodarone.

b. *Reduced effect*
Reduced absorption: cholestyramine
Increased metabolism: rifampicin, carbamazepine, griseofulvin, barbiturates.

2. Pharmacodynamic

a. *Enhanced effect*
   Liver damage: alcohol
   Increased catabolism of clotting factors: thyroxine
   Inhibition of clotting: heparin
   Inhibition of platelet function: aspirin and other NSAID, carbenicillin

b. *Reduced effect*
   Vitamin K (e.g. in parenteral nutrition)

THROMBOLYTIC AGENTS

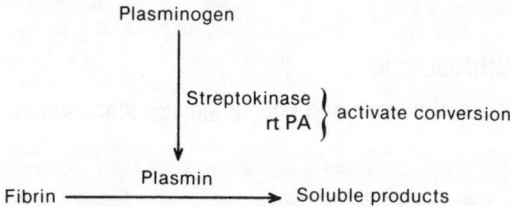

Plasminogen

Streptokinase }
           rt PA } activate conversion

Fibrin ⟶ Plasmin ⟶ Soluble products

Fig. 15.2

1. Streptokinase

Used in acute myocardial infarction in which it reduces mortality when given within the first 24 h. The earlier it is given the greater the benefit. Its efficacy is similar to that of aspirin and the two actions are additive. The two drugs are used together unless either is contraindicated. The adverse effects of streptokinase are of bleeding or are related to its immunogenicity. Contraindications include bleeding diathesis, active bleeding (e.g. from a peptic ulcer), recent surgical operation, post aggressive resuscitation (with chest massage), severe uncontrolled hypertension, recent stroke, recent streptococcal infection or treatment with streptokinase.

It is infused intravenously over 60 minutes and causes vasodilatation. A relative contraindication is therefore hypotension. A large clinical trial (ISIS III) showed it to be of similar efficacy to anistreplase and to alteplase. It is much less expensive than these two alternatives.

2. Anistreplase (anisoylated plasminogen streptokinase activator complex; APSAC).

Is effectively a streptokinase prodrug. Its efficacy in acute myocardial infarction is similar to streptokinase and gives rise to the same adverse effects, but is less likely to cause hypotension but rather more allergy and haemorrhage. It can be given as a relatively short

(5 minute) infusion. It is therefore possible that it will prove useful in very early myocardial infarction (pre-hospital), but it is more expensive than streptokinase.

3. Alteplase (recombinant tissue-type plasminogen activator; rt-PA). Is also effective in reducing mortality in acute myocardial infarction. Its beneficial effect requires subsequent administration of heparin to preserve patency of the opened vessel. It is not immunogenic, but can cause bleeding (including haemorrhagic stroke). It is much more expensive than streptokinase.

4. Urokinase
Has not been proven effective in myocardial infarction. It is currently used for thrombolysis in the eye (hyphaema). It is non-immunogenic.

INHIBITORS OF FIBRINOLYSIS

Inhibitors of plasminogen activation and encourage clot stabilisation.

Uses
Menorrhagia especially associated with IUD.
Haemorrhage, e.g. prostatectomy, post-dental extraction, peptic ulcer.
Sub-arachnoid haemorrhage — prevention of re-bleeding in acute phase.
Reversal of action of fibrinolytic drugs.

Drugs
Epsilon aminocaproic acid
— dose 3 g 4–6 times daily p.o.
Tranexamic acid
— dose 1 g 3–4 times daily p.o.
 or 1–2 g 3 times daily i.v. slowly.

ANTIPLATELET DRUGS

Reduce platelet aggregation. May prevent thromboembolism in atheroma and prosthetic heart valves. The only antiplatelet drug in routine clinical use of proven efficacy is aspirin.

Drug and dose	Action	Uses
Aspirin 300 mg on alternate days or 150 mg daily	Prevents platelet thromboxane generation; irreversible inhibition of prostaglandin synthetase. Reduction in thromboxane more long lasting than prostacyclin	Acute myocardial infarction. Secondary prevention following a myocardial infarction. Possibly primary prevention in individuals at high risk of myocardial infarction. Transient ischaemic attacks. Prevention of venous thrombosis. Prevention of emboli in atrial fibrillation. Prevention of graft occlusion following coronary artery grafting. Improved outcome of pregnancy in women at risk of pre-eclampsia
Dipyridamole	Inhibits adenosine uptake; inhibits platelet phosphodiesterase and raises platelet AMP levels	Uncertain efficacy. Used sometimes with aspirin after coronary artery bypass grafting. Also used with warfarin in patients with prosthetic valves
Epoprostenol (intravenous use only)	Raises platelet cAMP and inhibits aggregation	Cardiopulmonary bypass, haemodialysis when heparin is contraindicated
Ticlopidine	Inhibits fibrinogen binding to glycoprotein IIb/IIIa receptor	Of proven effectiveness in transient ischaemic attacks. Not in routine use because of severe neutropenia in a significant minority of patients

DISSEMINATED INTRAVASCULAR COAGULATION (DIC)

Many diseases can produce DIC.
1. Correct primary condition if possible.
2. Treat shock, blood loss, pH disturbances, hypoxia.
3. Give i.v. heparin if thrombosis in limb, pulmonary embolus or peripheral gangrene.
4. If bleeding, replace coagulation factors: e.g. platelets; fresh whole blood: fresh frozen plasma.
5. Inhibition of excessive fibrinolysis if lab tests show this with Epsilon-aminocaproic acid or Aprotinin.
Overall mortality is 50% — mainly due to underlying disease.

HAEMOLYTIC URAEMIC SYNDROME

Usually a child under the age of 3 years, over a week after an upper

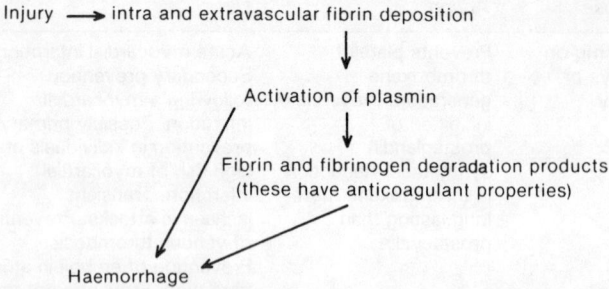

Injury ──→ intra and extravascular fibrin deposition
                              ↓
                    Activation of plasmin
                              ↓
                Fibrin and fibrinogen degradation products
                (these have anticoagulant properties)

        Haemorrhage

Fig. 15.3

respiratory or intestinal infection presents with anuria, anaemia and purpura. Untreated mortality is 30%. Treat with heparin plus peritoneal dialysis. Possible benefit with antiplatelet drugs.

BLEEDING IN LIVER DISEASE DUE TO LACK OF CLOTTING FACTORS

The following are synthesized in the liver:
  fibrinogen (factor I)
  factors V, XI, XII, XIII
  factors II, VII, IX, X (vitamin K dependent)
  plasminogen
  fibrinolytic inhibitors
  coagulation inhibitors.

Obstructive jaundice
Coagulation defect corrected by parenteral vitamin K.

Acute liver failure
Bleeding because of DIC plus lack of clotting factors.

Chronic liver disease
Can result in DIC, thrombocytopenia, lack of fibrinogen and a readily lysed clot. If haemorrhage occurs or surgery is to be performed vitamin K is given parenterally plus fresh frozen plasma (up to 1 litre). Platelet infusions may be given in addition.

HAEMOPHILIA

Haemophilia A — congenital bleeding disorder inherited as sex-linked disorder producing factor VIII activity deficiency in plasma.

Haemophilia B (Christmas disease) — similar inheritance and clinical features to haemophilia B but due to lack of factor IX.

Von Willebrand's disease — congenital bleeding disorder inherited as autosomal dominant. Patients have prolonged bleeding time, abnormal platelet function and reduced level of factor VIII activity. Factor VIII: not stable at room temperature; in vivo $T_{\frac{1}{2}} = 6-8$ h. Factor IX: not stable at room temperature; in vivo $T_{\frac{1}{2}} = 12-15$ h.

The treatment of a bleeding episode is intravenous replacement of clotting factors. For a haemarthrosis, infusion is for 4–6 h and clotting factor levels raised to 20–30% of normal. However visceral or intra-abdominal haemorrhage requires bed rest and clotting factors to be raised to 50%. For surgical operation infusions are continued until 10 days afterwards and during the procedure the deficient clotting factor is raised to normal levels. The concentrates used are:

Cryoprecipitate — stored frozen. Rapidly thawed at 37°C in 200–300 ml batches and used immediately by infusion over a 30 minute period.

Factor VIII and IX concentrates — stored in lyophilised form and diluted with water and then immediately injected (usually volumes of 50–100 ml).

These products from donor blood have allowed the transmission of HIV. The cryoprecipitate (and other similar products) are now highly purified and sterilized by heat. Genetically engineered clotting factors are not yet generally available.

Desmopressin (DDAVP) given by intravenous infusion is used in patients with von Willebrand's disease before elective surgical procedures.

IRON

Average Western diet contains 10–20 mg iron.

ABSORPTION

Daily intestinal absorption 1 mg (males), 2 mg (females). Ferrous iron absorbed more readily than ferric iron. Enhancement of absorption by: low pH of intestinal contents; high protein diet; ascorbic acid; potentiated mucosal transport (as in iron deficiency and increased erythropoiesis).

ADMINISTRATION

Oral iron
Iron deficiency — first exclude blood loss. Replace with: ferrous sulphate 100–200 mg orally daily (in divided doses) continuing for 6 months to provide reserve stores. Repeat blood picture after the first month (haemoglobin should rise by 0.1 g/dL/day).

Others: ferrous fumarate, gluconate and succinate absorbed as well as sulphate. Sustained-release preparations should not be used. Liquid preparations are used in small children in the form of ferrous glycine sulphate or sodium ironedetate elixir. The use of a dropper may avoid staining of the teeth.

Toxicity
Consists of GI upset (20–30%) — ferrous iron irritates mucosa causing nausea, discomfort and bowel disturbance. Try changing preparation; reducing dose; giving with food (but may reduce absorption).

Parenteral iron
Only justified if patient unable to take oral iron. Can cause fever, arthralgia, anaphylaxis.

Contraindications to iron
Risk of iron overload and siderosis if iron given unnecessarily in:
haemolytic ⎫
hypoplastic ⎬ anaemia
sideroblastic ⎭
renal failure
anaemia of chronic inflammation
thalassaemia.

FOLIC ACID

(= pteroylglutamic acid.) Activated in the body to 5-methyltetrahydrolate, which acts as a 1C donor for several metabolic reactions including synthesis of purine and pyrimidine bases and interconversions of aminoacids. Folate deficiency results in megaloblastic anaemia.

Pharmacokinetics
Daily requirement (100–150 µg) usually supplied in normal diet (100–200 µg). Absorbed in duodenum and jejunum, with no limitation on rate on transmucosal absorption. An enterohepatic circulation is present. Loose binding to plasma albumin. Body stores (10–15 mg) last for 4 months. Normal serum folate 3.0–15.0 µg/l; RBC folate 145–450 µg/l.

Administration
Care to exclude vitamin B_{12} deficiency before starting. Oral folic acid 5 mg daily is initial treatment.

VITAMIN B_{12}

(= a group of cobalamins, including methyl cobalamin and

deoxyadenosyl cobalamin. Hydroxycobalamin is used in treatment). It is in foods of primary animal origin. A mixed diet supplies 5 µg/day; a vegetarian diet contains 0.5 µg — mainly from milk and bacterial contamination of food. The daily need is 1–2 µg/day.

Vitamin B_{12} deficiency causes an arrest in folate metabolism by:
a. blocking demethylation of methyltetrahydrofolate,
b. failure of entry of folate into cells.

Vitamin B_{12} is needed for the synthesis of methionine and the conversion of methylmalonic acid to succinic acid.

Pharmacokinetics
Maximum daily absorption capacity (2 µg) is daily requirement. Absorption in ileum in presence of intrinsic factor. Bound in plasma to transcobalamin II. Enterohepatic circulation is present. Body stores (2–4 mg) last 3–4 yrs. Normal serum levels 170–1000 µg/l.

Administration
Treatment of megaloblastic anaemia due to vitamin B_{12} deficiency is injections of hydroxycobalamin, 250 µg every 4–8 weeks for life.

Response to treatment (Vitamin B_{12} or folate)
Subjective improvement 24–48 h
Normoblastic marrow 48 h
Start of reticulocyte response 3 days
Peak of reticulocyte response 6 days
Hb normal 6 weeks.

ADVERSE HAEMATOLOGICAL RESPONSE TO DRUGS

1. *Cytotoxic agents*
   produce dose-dependent depression of all marrow elements (i.e. aplastic anaemia).

2. *Idiosyncratic agranulocytosis:*
   phenylbutazone and oxyphenylbutazone
   chloramphenicol
   amidopyrines
   sulphonamides and dapsone
   phenothiazines
   antithyroid drugs
   captopril.

3. *Idiosyncratic aplastic anaemia:*
   phenylbutazone and oxyphenylbutazone
   chloramphenicol
   phenothiazines
   phenytoin and troxidone
   sodium aurothiomalate.

4. *Idiosyncractic thrombocytopenia:*
   quinidine and quinine
   phenylbutazone and oxyphenylbutazone
   thiazides
   heparin
   gold
   chloramphenicol.

5. *Anaemia:*
   dyshaemopoietic, e.g. folate deficiency due to methotrexate or
                     phenytoin. Trimethoprim and pyrimethamine
                     can contribute to folate deficiency.
                     Prolonged nitrous oxide anaesthesia leads
                     to anaemia by degrading enzyme-bound
                     vitamin B_{12}.
   haemolytic, e.g. methyldopa
                   G6PD deficiency plus primaquine
                   penicillin
   haemorrhagic, e.g. NSAID
   aplasia, e.g. chloramphenicol.

Management of aplastic anaemia
1. Remove cause, if suspected.
2. Support with blood products and treat infections.
3. Specific therapy:
   corticosteroids
   androgens (oxymetholone; etiocholanolone)
   marrow transplantation
   antithymocyte globulin
   antilymphocyte globulin.

16. Hormones and drugs acting on the endocrine system

ANTERIOR PITUITARY HORMONES

Growth hormone (GH)
Prolactin
Gonadotrophins (FSH and LH)
Corticotrophin (ACTH)

POSTERIOR PITUITARY HORMONES

Vasopressin
Oxytocin

ANTERIOR PITUITARY

Growth hormone (GH) is species-specific

Actions
1. Potentiates protein synthesis.
2. Synergistic effect with insulin in increasing flow of amino acids into cells.
3. Stimulates somatomedin secretion by liver which mediates skeletal growth.

Use of GH
Only indication is growth failure in children due to GH lack. GH from human pituitaries can transmit Creutzfeldt–Jakob dementia.
Genetically engineered GH (somatropin) is now used instead.

Prolactin
Hyperprolactinaemia
→ infertility, amenorrhoea, galactorrhoea in women.
→ hypogonadism, impotence, gynaecomastia in men.
Increased secretion: dopamine antagonists (neuroleptics; metoclopramide).
Decreased secretion: dopamine agonists (dopamine; bromocriptine).

Bromocriptine
Dopamine receptor agonist which reduces prolactin secretion.

Uses
1. Suppression of puerperal lactation: 2.5 mg initially followed by 2.5 mg twice daily for 2 weeks. Residual breast tenderness: given 2.5 mg daily for a further week.
2. Hyperprolactinaemia associated with infertility and hypogonadism: 2.5–7.5 mg twice daily for 2–6 months. Stop treatment (in females) if pregnancy occurs. Pituitary tumours may expand, thus measure visual fields.
3. Cyclical benign breast disease.
4. Acromegaly.
5. Parkinsonism — see section on neurological disease.

Toxicity
Constipation
Nausea, vomiting
Giddiness, hypotension and fainting
Cramps
Dystonia
Hallucinations.

Table 29 Stimulation of ovulation

Drug	Action	Use
Clomiphene Cyclofenil Tamoxifen	Anti-oestrogen which blocks oestrogen receptors in hypothalamus and thus causes release of FSH and LH, which in turn stimulates ovulation and formation of corpus luteum	Main indication is infertile female, esp. with secondary amenorrhoea
FSH (with LH)	Additional gonadotrophin	Infertility due to hypopituitarism when higher doses of clomiphene have not produced ovulation. *Toxicity:* multiple pregnancy, raised abortion rate, ovarian enlargement
Bromocriptine	Dopamine agonist. Dopamine inhibits prolactin secretion. Thus bromocriptine will correct hyperprolactinaemia	Infertility associated with hyperprolactinaemia (when thyroid and pituitary diseases have been excluded). Drug is stopped as soon as pregnancy occurs

Gonadotrophins
FSH

— Controls development of primary ovarian follicle; stimulates granulosa cell proliferation; increases oestrogen secretion } females
— increases spermatogenesis   — males

LH

— Produces ovulation; stimulates thecal oestrogen secretion; initiates and maintains corpus luteum } females
— stimulates androgen secretion from Leydig cells.   — males

FSH is used for female infertility which has not responded to clomiphene. It is used with LH. *Menotrophin* contains FSH and LH; *urofollitrophin* has FSH; *chorionic gonadotrophin* has LH activity. Treatment is carefully monitored to reduce the risk of multiple pregnancy.

Danazol
Inhibits gonadotrophin secretion from the pituitary. It has androgenic, antioestrogen and antiprogestogen effects. It is used in the treatment of endometriosis and some menstrual and breast abnormalities.

Cestrinone
An alternative to danazol in the treatment of endometriosis. It reduces gonadotrophin secretion and decreases levels of sex hormone-binding globulin.

Clomiphene
Blocks oestrogen receptors in the hypothalamus and thus increases secretion of gonadotrophin releasing hormone. Thus induces ovulation in polycystic ovary syndrome and in post pill amenorrhoea.

Corticosteroids
Suppress hypothalamic and pituitary secretion. Used for this property in idiopathic hirsutes and in hirsutes in the polycystic ovary syndrome.

Octeotride
A synthetic analogue of somatostatin. It inhibits secretion of alimentary endocrine tumours and is used for the treatment of vipoma, glucagonoma and carcinoid.

POSTERIOR PITUITARY

Oxytocin and Vasopressin
Synthesised in anterior hypothalamic nuclei and travel in nerve fibres to posterior lobe of pituitary.

Oxytocin
Octapeptide.
Produces contraction of uterus and mammary gland ducts.

Kinetics
Destroyed by trypsin.
Absorbed from buccal and nasal mucosae but given by i.v. infusion
$T\frac{1}{2}$ = 5–10 mins (but action more prolonged).

Uses
1. Initiation and augmentation of labour.
2. Post partum haemorrhage and management of 3rd stage of labour:
   oxytocin given with ergometrine.

Toxicity
1. Excessive action (uterine rupture; fetal asphyxia).
2. Water retention and intoxication, hypertension with large doses.

   Other agents used to stimulate the uterus include prostaglandins:
dinoprost to induce abortion and *carboprost* for uterine atony in the
3rd stage of labour.

Vasopressin (antidiuretic hormone; ADH)
Similar octapeptide structure to oxytocin.

Secretion
Increased by:
raised plasma osmotic pressure
decreased blood volume
emotional and physical stress
morphine, nicotine.

Actions
1. Increases water reabsorption by distal renal tubules and collecting
   ducts.
2. Vasoconstriction.

Kinetics
Similar to oxytocin — can be administered by injection or nasal
insufflation.

Uses
1. Vasopressin or terlipressin are infused intravenously to treat
   bleeding oesophageal varices.
2. In cranial diabetes insipidus:
   a. Pig or beef vasopressin injections effective for 3–5 hours.
      Vasopressin snuff effective but allergenic and therefore
      obsolescent.

b. Synthetic lysine vasopressin — lypressin — nasal spray for mild diabetes insipidus but short lasting. No local or pulmonary complications: Plasma $T_{1/2}$ = 15 mins. Metered dose 3–7 times daily.

c. 1-desamino-8-D-arginine vasopressin — desmopressin (DDAVP) — Synthetic long-acting analogue or vasopressin. $T_{1/2}$ = 75 mins. Administered i.v. or i.m or intranasally once or twice daily. No local or pulmonary toxicity. At present drug of choice for diabetes insipidus. Also used for enuresis.

d. In mild diabetes insipidus: chlorpropamide (increases renal sensitivity to vasopressin); carbamazepine (increases vasopressin secretion); demeclocycline also used.

e. Thiazide diuretics used in nephrogenic diabetes insipidus.

ADRENAL CORTICOSTEROIDS
Secretions of adrenal cortex:
1. Glucocorticoids: cortisol and corticosterone
2. Mineralocorticoids: aldosterone and small amounts of desoxycorticosterone.
3. Small amounts of testosterone, androsterone, oestrogens, progesterone.

Uses of systemic steroids

Replacement
Addison's disease and other forms of adrenal cortical insufficiency.
Hypopituitarism

Anti-inflammatory
Rheumatic disorders
Allergic reactions
Immunosuppression (e.g. organ transplantation, collagen diseases)
Specific clinical problems (e.g. severe asthma).

Suppression of ACTH
Congenital adrenal hyperplasia.

Local steroid treatment is used to avoid or reduce systemic toxicity e.g. intra articular, inhaled, skin application, eye drops, enemas.

Chronic hypoadrenalism
1. Oral hydrocortisone — 20 mg morning + 10 mg evening (prednisolone is an alternative).
2. More severely affected: add fludrocortisone 0.05–0.2 mg/day.
3. Intercurrent illness:
   — mild: double cortisol dose
   — moderate: i.m. or i.v. hydrocortisone 100 mg 6-hourly.

Table 30 Actions of cortisol and consequences of under- and over-secretion

	Actions	Deficiency	Excess
Carbohydrate, protein and fat metabolism	Enhances gluconeogenesis; antagonises insulin hypoglycaemia ± diabetes mellitus; centripetal fat disposition; hypertriglyceridaemia; hypercholesterolaemia; decreased protein synthesis, e.g. diminished skin collagen	Hypoglycaemia Loss of weight	Cushing's syndrome. Weight gain; increase in trunk fat; moon face; skin striae; bruising; atrophy wasting of limb muscles
Water and salt metabolism	Inhibits fluid shift from extracellular into intra cellular compartment; antagonises vasopressin action on kidney; increases vasopressin destruction and decreases its production. Sodium and water retention, potassium loss	Loss of weight Hypovolaemia Hyponatraemia	Oedema; thirst; polyuria. Hypertension. Muscular weakness
Haematological	Lowers lymphocyte and eosinophil counts; increases RBC, platelets and clotting tendency		Florid complexion and polycythaemia
Alimentary	Increased production of gasric acid and pepsin	Anorexia and nausea	Dyspepsia
CVS	Sensitises arterioles to catecholamines enhances production of angiotensinogen. Fall in high density lipoprotein with increased total cholesterol	Hypotension Fainting	Hypertension Atherosclerosis
Skeletal	Decreased production of cartilage and bone; osteoporosis; anti-vitamin D; increased renal loss of calcium; renal calculi formation		Backache due to osteoporosis Renal calculi Dwarfing in children (also anti-GH effect)

Table 30 (continued)

	Actions	Deficiency	Excess
Nervous system	Altered neuronal excitability. Inhibition of uptake$_2$ of catecholamines		Depression and other psychiatric changes
Anti-inflammatory	Reduces formation of fluid and cellular exudate; reduces fibrous tissue repair		Increased spread of and proneness to infections
Immunological	Large doses lyse lymphocytes and plasma cells (transient release of immunoglobulin)		Reduced lymphocyte mass Diminished immunoglobulin production
Feedback	Inhibits release of ACTH and MSH. Growth arrest may be due to inhibition of growth hormone release	Pigmentation of skin and mucosa	

4. Surgery: i.m. or i.v. hydrocortisone 100 mg 6-hourly, from 2 hours before operation till oral feeding resumed.

Acute hypoadrenalism
1. i.v. 0.9% NaCl + glucose (enough to maintain fluid and salt balance and blood glucose).
2. i.v. cortisol (hydrocortisone hemisuccinate) 100 mg 6-hourly or more frequently (enough to maintain BP).
3. When electrolyte balance restored and vomiting stopped, give oral cortisol 20 mg 6-hourly initially then reduce.
   Mineralocorticoid may have to be introduced with lower doses of cortisol.

Pituitary deficiency
Oral hydrocortisone needed but not usually mineralocorticoids.
Thyroxine and sex hormones given according to need.

Some important examples of anti-inflammatory uses of glucocorticoids
Temporal arteritis (giant cell arteritis) and polymyalgia rheumatica
Myasthenia gravis (esp. failed thymectomy; patients unsuitable for thymectomy)
Dermatomyositis and polymyositis
Infantile salaam attacks with hypsarrhythmia
Reduction of oedema around tumours (esp. mediastinum; intracranial)

Table 31 Relative activities of glucocorticoids and mineralocorticoids

Drug	Compared with cortisol (w/w) Mineralocorticoid activity	Glucocorticoid and anti-inflammatory activity	Special features	Equivalent dose for anti-inflammatory effect (mg)
Cortisol	1	1	$T_{1/2} = 2$ h (but biological effects $T_{1/2} = 12$ h)	20
Cortisone	Inactive but converted to cortisol in liver	×4		25
Prednisolone	×0.8		$T_{1/2} = 2.5–3$ h (but biological effects $T_{1/2} = 12$ h). Mainly used for anti-inflammatory actions	5
Prednisone	Inactive but converted to prednisolone in liver			5
Methylprednisolone	×0.5	×5		4
Triamcinolone (9-α-fluoro-16-α-hydroxy prednisolone)	0	×5	Can produces flushes, sweating and muscular weakness. Arthritis on withdrawal. Plus glucocorticoid side-effects. Used as an anti-inflammatory	4
Betamethasone	0	×25	Used for anti-inflammatory actions and to suppress corticotrophin release	0.75
Dexamethasone	0	×25		
Fludrocortisone	×125	×10	Used for its mineralocorticoid activity in hypoadrenal states	—
Aldosterone	×1000	0	Has to be injected. Not used clinically	—

Severe bronchial asthma and bronchitis
Pulmonary sarcoidosis
Pulmonary alveolitis (allergic and fibrosing)
Minimal change nephrotic syndrome
SLE; polyarteritis nodosa
Angioedema; anaphylaxis
Acquired haemolytic anaemia
Acute leukaemias (lymphocytolytic action)
Rheumatic fever
Chronic active hepatitis
Ulcerative colitis
Crohn's disease
Exfoliative dermatitis; pemphigus.

TESTIS

Main hormone is testosterone, secreted by interstitial (Leydig) cells.
Testosterone is anabolic and causes masculinisation. In *normal* males
it depresses spermatogenesis and inhibits release of pituitary
gonadotrophins.

Uses
Androgens are useless in the treatment of primary impotence, but in
hypopituitarism can lead to normal sexual development and potency.
Fertility and spermatogenesis are not restored and menotrophin (FSH)
plus LH or chorionic gonadotrophin have to be added to promote
spermatogenesis in hypopituitary states.

Gonadal deficiency is treated with androgens, but in children with
delayed puberty premature fusion of epiphyses can be caused.

Some oestrogen-dependent breast cancers and metastases regress
with androgens.

Administration
Testosterone or its esters can be given as a depot injection
intramuscularly.

Mesterolone is active orally. Methyltestosterone, like other 17 α
alkyl steroids, can cause cholestatic jaundice.

Anabolic steroids
Nandrolone and stanozolol have some androgenic action but are less
virilising in the female than testosterone.

No beneficial effect has been proved in osteoporosis wasting
diseases, body building and in athletics. They are used in some
aplastic anaemias and to reduce itch in chronic biliary obstruction.

The anabolic steroids can cause headache, mood change and
premature epiphyseal fusion. The 17 α alkyl derivatives may produce
jaundice.

Cyproterone

An anti-androgen with progestogenic properties. Used to suppress sexual activity in men with unacceptable sexual behaviour and to treat acne and hirsutism in women.

OESTROGENS

Oestrogens are necessary for the development of female secondary sex characteristics, including uterine musculature and cornification of the vaginal epithelium. In doses used for contraception they suppress ovulation and inhibit the release of FSH.

Oral oestrogens undergo high first pass metabolism but transdermal patch administration gives a more physiological pattern of delivery.

Ethinyl oestradiol and conjugated oestrogens are widely used. Oestradiol is available in a self-adherent plaster. Tibolone (used in HRT) has additional progestogenic and androgenic actions, and does not have to be given with cyclical progestogens.

Uses

1. In combined contraceptive pill.
2. Replacement in hypofunctioning ovary (menopause and primary amenorrhoea).
3. Carcinoma of prostate (and some breast carcinomas).
4. Functional uterine haemorrhage.

Specific indications in climacteric

Prevention of osteoporosis — esp. with strong family history or other predisposing factors
Vasomotor instability
Lower genital tract atrophy.

Toxicity

Nausea
Breast tenderness
Vaginal discharge
Leg cramps
Weight gain, sodium and water retention
Raised blood pressure
Endometrial hyperplasia and carcinoma (incidence reduced by adding progestogens to regime)
Thromboembolism.

Contraindications to oestrogen treatment

Absolute contraindications — breast carcinoma
— endometrial hyperplasia or carcinoma or undiagnosed vaginal bleeding.

Myocardial infarction
Stroke or other thromboembolic disease
Porphyria
Hyperlipoproteinaemia
Pregnancy
Obesity
Heavy smoker
Hypertension
Active liver disease
Breast dysplasia.

PROGESTOGENS

Act principally on reproductive organs.

Unlike oestrogens and androgens, have few systemic effects but synthetic progestogens variably metabolised to oestrogens and androgens.

Act mainly on tissues sensitised by oestrogens but effects inhibited by oestrogens.

Naturally occuring: progesterone and analogues (e.g. dydrogesterone)
Testosterone-derived progestogens: e.g. norethisterone.

Uses
1. Contraception.
2. With oestrogens given for long term hormone replacement.
3. Dysmenorrhoea — given on days 20–25 of cycle (oral contraceptives to suppress ovulation are effective).
4. Endometriosis — prolonged doses of progestogens or oral contraceptives with high progestogen content.
5. Functional uterine haemorrhage — induce regular bleeding with oral contraceptives or give progestogen on 20–25 days of cycle.

ORAL CONTRACEPTIVES

Despite their important social consequences and convenience these are potent drugs and because they are used in well women safety must be paramount.

Three main types
1. *Combination:* one oestrogen/progestogen tablet daily for 21 days starting on day 7 of menstrual cycle, repeated after 7 pill-free days. Maximum oestrogen dose now 50 μg/day.
2. *Triphasic formulations* which more closely mimic endogenous cyclic hormonal activity, e.g. Logynon, Trinordiol. Beginning on first day of period daily regime is:

Days	Content of each pill (μg)	
	Ethinyloestradiol	Levonorgestrel
1–6	30	50
7–11	40	75
12–21	30	125
22–28	No pill taken	

Efficacy and use of this formulation not established.
3. *Progestogen only* — continuous administration of progestogen one tablet daily starting on day 1 of period.

Pharmacology
1. Oestrogen-progestogen combined pill acts at several levels:
   a. Oestrogen inhibits FSH release and progestogen inhibits midcycle LH surge required for ovulation.
   b. Ovarian steroidogenesis (especially progestogen) inhibited.
   c. Endometrial changes make implantation less likely.
   d. Cervical mucus remains thick and impermeable to sperm at ovulation.
   e. ? interferes with coordinated contractions of cervix and fallopian tubes important for sperm transport.

   Abrupt withdrawal of progestogen at the end of each dose interval (21 days) results in withdrawal uterine bleeding like a period.
2. Progestogen only pill — main actions on cervical mucus and endometrium to prevent fertilisation and implantation. Inhibits ovulation (in 40% women). Success rate lower than combined pill. Menstruation occurs despite continuous progestogen administration but bleeding less predictable and duration variable.

Other important pharmacological effects
1. Enhanced blood clotting due to:
   a. increased platelet aggregation
   b. decreased antithrombin III
   c. increased clotting factors
   d. decreased plasminogen activator in vessel walls.
2. Hypertension (? due to increased renin substrate synthesis) — usually resolved 6 months after discontinuation.
3. Decreased glucose tolerance.
4. Cholestatic jaundice (especially if history of pregnancy jaundice).
5. Secondary amenorrhoea and infertility after stopping pill.

Pharmacokinetics
Natural oestrogens and progestogens undergo extensive first-pass metabolism and are ineffective orally so synthetic oestrogens (ethinyloestradiol or its methoxy analogue mestranol used) and progestogens (19-nortestosterone derivatives — levonorgestrel, norethisterone and ethynodiol) used. 19-nortestosterone derivatives

can have some androgenic action and also metabolised to oestrogens (may account for anti-ovulatory effect in some women).

Undergo hepatic metabolism and enterohepatic recirculation — broad spectrum antibiotics inhibit gut flora which release hormone from glucuronide for reabsorption.

Drug interactions
Contraceptive failure possible if inducing agents given, e.g. phenytoin, carbamazepine, phenobarbitone, rifampicin, or gut flora altered by antibiotic, e.g. ampicillin.

Absolute contraindications
1. Thrombophlebitis, thromboembolic disorders, CVS disease, coronary artery disease (and past history of these).
2. Significantly impaired liver function.
3. Known or suspected breast cancer.
4. Known or suspected oestrogen-dependent neoplasm.
5. Undiagnosed cause of vaginal bleeding.
6. Known or suspected pregnancy.

Increased risk of CVS disease if pill used in patients with
1. Hyperlipidaemia (especially type IIa)
2. Diabetes mellitus
3. Hypertension; previous hypertension of pregnancy
4. Obesity
5. Tobacco smoking
6. Progressive rise in risk over age 30 — especially with high oestrogen use for prolonged period
7. Family history of MI, cerebrovascular disease or pulmonary embolism before age of 50.

NB: Risk may persist after stopping Pill (? how long).

Increased risk of thrombophlebitis
1. Varicose veins
2. Obesity.

Other contraindications to pill
Cholelithiasis (increased frequency of gall stones on pill)
Multiple sclerosis
Porphyria (precipitates acute attack).

Toxicity of pill

A. *Symptoms and signs*	*Pill must be stopped because possible cause is:*
Blindness, proptosis, diplopia, papilloedema	Retinal artery thrombosis

Unilateral or central chest pain or tingling. Pains or weakness in arms. Haemoptysis. Dyspnoea	Myocardial infarction; pulmonary embolism
Leg pains, tenderness or swelling	Thrombophlebitis
Slurring of speech	Stroke
Hepatic mass or tenderness	Liver neoplasm

B.	*Pill may be continued only if the following are excluded:*
Amenorrhoea	Pregnancy
Breakthrough bleeding	Genital cancer
Breast lumps, pain, swelling	Breast carcinoma
Right upper abdominal pain	Cholecystitis, cholelithiasis, liver cancer
Mid epigastric pain	Abdominal artery or vein thrombosis, pulmonary embolism, myocardial infarction
Migraine	Vascular spasm preceding a cerebral thrombosis
Non-migraine headache	Hypertension
Jaundice; itching	Cholestatic jaundice
Increase in uterine size	Uterine tumour; adenomyosis; pregnancy

C. Toxicity due to oestrogen excess:
Increased serum proteins (including clotting factors, steroid and thyroid binding proteins, renin substrate, caeruloplasmin)
Hypertriglyceridaemia
Vascular: thromboembolic disease, migraine, myocardial infarction, stroke (increased 6–8 times)
Skin: cloasma, telangiectasia, capillary fragility
Gynaecological: vaginal mucous discharge, uterine enlargement and leiomyomas, excessive uterine blood loss
Breasts: cystic breast hypertrophy.

D. Toxicity due to progestogen excess:
CNS: tiredness, depression, decreased libido, increased appetite and weight gain
CVS: dilated leg veins; decreased high density lipoprotein cholesterol (therefore possible increase in atheroma)
Skin: oily skin and scalp, acne, neurodermatitis
Gynaecological: pelvic congestion, cervicitis, moniliasis, scanty periods
Breasts: tenderness, increased alveolar mass
Liver: jaundice.

C plus D
Hypertension

E. Fluid retention effects
Due to oestrogen excess if occur on pill days and progestogen excess if occur on pill-free days: nausea and vomiting; dizziness and syncope; oedema; leg cramps; irritability; bloating cyclic weight gain; headaches or visual disturbances.

F. Relative oestrogen deficiency
Breakthrough bleeding days 1–7
Continuous breakthrough bleeding
Scanty or absent menstruation
Nervousness
Vasomotor symptoms
Dysparunia due to dry vagina.

G. Relative progestogen deficiency
Breakthrough bleeding days 8–21
Heavy menstruation and/or delayed menstruation
Dysmenorrhoea
Weight loss.

Mortality

Mortality per 100 000 women aged 35–49
Oral contraceptive users — 3.9
Non pill users — 0.5
Risk of dying during pregnancy — 58
Risk of dying due to thromboembolism during pregnancy — 2.3
Mortality in pill users mainly consequences of thromboembolism (blood group O pill users have ⅓ this risk).

Morbidity versus Efficacy

Method of contraception	Excess of admissions to hospital (per 100 women years)		Pregnancies (per 100 women years)
Pill	Stroke	0.035	0.36
	Thromboembolic disease	0.07	
	MI	0.01	
IUD	Uterine perforation	0.05	2.0
	Pelvic inflammatory disease	0.2	
Occlusive devices	NIL		5.0

INSULIN

INSULIN

Proinsulin synthesized in β-cells of islets; C-peptide cleaved off in storage granules to form insulin. At secretion equivalent amounts of insulin and C-peptide released into blood.

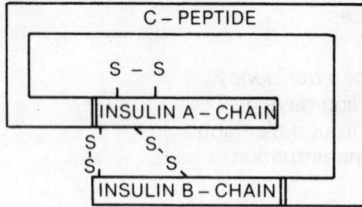

```
                    ┌────────────────────────────────┐
                    │          C – PEPTIDE            │
                    │  ┌──────────────────────────┐   │
                    │  │         S – S            │   │
                    │  │ ║INSULIN A – CHAIN        │   │
                    │  S    S                     │   │
                    │  S│   S  S                   │   │
                    │  ║INSULIN B – CHAIN║         │   │
                    └────────────────────────────────┘
```

Fig. 16.1

Blood insulin and C-peptide high when glucose is given. Endogenous insulin and C-peptide low when insulin is administered.
Diabetic state (diabetus mellitus; DM) is a sustained and abnormal elevation of blood glucose concentration which is due to a relative or absolute deficiency of insulin action.

  Most insulin used in treatment is pig or of human sequence. Antigenicity mainly due to C-peptide and other non insulin peptides. Thus antigenicity is low in highly purified (monocomponent) insulins in which these have been removed.

Actions of insulin
1. Increased glucose uptake by muscle and fat.
2. Inhibition of gluconeogenesis.
3. Conversion of glucose to glycogen and fatty acids promoted.
4. Conversion of fatty acids to triglycerides promoted and reverse reactions inhibited.
5. Conversion of aminoacids to proteins promoted and reverse reactions inhibited.

Pharmacokinetics
Insulin polypeptide destroyed by gut enzymes and so given parenterally. T½ is 6–10 mins but various pharmaceutical processes can produce products with different absorption characteristics and therefore different durations of action.

HUMAN INSULIN

Two types:
1. Semi-synthetic — chemical substitution of the alanine at B30 of porcine insulin by threonine (emp).

— Human Actrapid
— Human Monotard
2. Total synthesis of A and B chains separately by recombinant DNA techniques using *E. coli* which are then combined into biosynthetic human insulin (crb, prb, pyr).
— Humulin S (like soluble insulin)
— Humulin I (like isophane insulin)
    Effects similar to animal insulins. Early hopes that it would be non-allergenic have not been fulfilled. The onset of action is more rapid and abrupt which poses the danger of hypoglycaemia when changing from porcine to human insulin.

Indications for insulin
1. DM with ketosis or polyuria and weight loss. Usually but not always present under 30.
2. DM not adequately controlled with diet and oral agent. Any complications.
3. Hyperglycaemic ketoacidosis.
4. Critical episodes in DM, e.g. operations, infections, ischaemia, trauma and pregnancy.

Clinical use
1. New patients started on highly purified MC insulins.
2. Most satisfactory regime is multiple dosing (single dosing with long acting insulins in elderly, visually disabled and those needing < 30 IU/day).
    a. Start with 2 injections of soluble insulin before breakfast and supper.
    b. If saw-tooth pattern of glycaemia then replace part or whole of one or both doses with intermediate acting insulin.
    c. If further smoothing needed, then a long acting insulin given before supper plus 2 or more injections of short acting insulin during the day.
    d. During childbirth, crises and in brittle diabetes closed or open loop systems (artificial pancreas) may be used.
3. Reduce insulin dose if unusual activity undertaken or if food consumption is reduced.

Toxicity of insulin
1. Hypoglycaemia
2. Post-hypoglycaemic hyperglycaemia (Somogyi effect)
3. Local and systemic allergy (uncommon)
4. Insulin resistance due to insulin antibodies
5. Acquired increased susceptibility to insulin
6. Lipodystrophy (becoming less common with use of purified insulins).

Table 32 Insulin preparations

Type of insulin	Proprietary preparation	Type of insulin	Onset of activity (h)	Peak activity (h)	Duration of activity (h)
1. Rapidly acting, short duration					
Insulin BP (Soluble insulin)	Soluble	Solution. Beef	1	3–5	6–8
Neutral insulin BP	Hypurin Neutral	Highly purified. Beef	½	2–6	6–8
	Actrapid MC	Monocomponent. Pork	1	3–5	7
	Velosulin (Leo Neutral)	Highly purified. Pork	1	1½–3½	7–8
	Nuso (neutral soluble)	Solution. Beef	1	3–5	6–8
2. Intermediate duration of action					
Isophane insulin BP (Isophane protamine insulin)	Insulatard (Leo Retard)	Highly purified crystalline suspension. Pork	2	4–12	24
	Isophane NPH	Crystalline suspension. Beef	2½	5–14	18–27
Insulin zinc suspension (amorphous) BP	Semitard MC	Monocomponent amorphous suspension. Pork.	1½	4–10	16
	Semilente	Amorphous suspension. Pork	1	4–8	12–16
Globin zinc insulin BP	Globin	Crystalline suspension. Pork	2	6–12	18–24
3. Long duration of action					
Insulin zinc suspension (crystalline) BP	Ultratard MC	Monocomponent crystalline suspension. Beef.	4	10–30	35
	Ultralente	Crystalline suspension	4–8	10–30	30–35

Table 32 (continued)

Type of insulin	Proprietary preparation	Type of insulin	Onset of activity (h)	Peak activity (h)	Duration of activity (h)
Protamine zinc insulin BP	Hypurin protamine zinc	Highly purified suspension. Beef. Contains excess protamine and zinc.	4–6	10–20	24–35
	Protamine Zinc Insulin (PZI)	Amorphous suspension. Beef. Contains an excess of protamine and zinc	4–8	10–20	24–34
4. Mixed preparations					
Biphasic insulin BP	Rapitard MC	Monocomponent. Mixed beef and pork. Suspension of 25% Actrapid MC and 75% crystalline	1½	4–12	22
	Mixtard 30/70 (Leo Mixtard)	Highly purified. Pork. 30% Velosulin and 70% of Insulatard	½	2–8	24
Insulin zinc suspension BP (insulin zinc suspension (mixed))	Monotard MC	Monocomponent. Pork. Suspension of 30% amorphous and 70% crystalline	3	6½–14	22
	Lentard MC	Monocomponent. Mixed beef and pork. Suspension of 30% amorphous and 70% crystalline	3	6½–14	24
	Lente	Beef suspension of 30% amorphous and 70% crystalline	2½	6–14	22–29

Comas in diabetics

Type	Management
Hyperglycaemic with ketoacidosis	See Table 33
Hyperglycaemic without ketosis	See Table 33
Hypoglycaemic	*Prevent:* care with different insulin strengths; patient takes meal or glucose tablets when early symptoms appear. 20 ml of 10% glucose i.v. usually successful *or* 1 mg of glucagon i.m. i.v. injection of 50% glucose not usually required.
Lactic acidosis	i.v. fluids containing bicarbonate. Dialyse.
Renal failure	Renal failure regime including dialysis, treatment of encephalopathy, correction of electrolyte disturbances.

Diet in diabetes

1. Patient education — including spacing of meals, relationship of food and hypoglycaemic agents, lipids and atheroma, recognition of hyper and hypoglycaemia.
2. Initial dietary trial for 4 weeks in order to assess whether symptoms, 2 h post prandial hyperglycaemia (<13–14 mmol/l) and ketonuria can be readily controlled by diet alone.
3. If patient is obese restrict calories and increase exercise to attain ideal weight. Fat must be restricted more than carbohydrate.
Calorie needs:
inactive — ideal body weight (lbs) × 10
sedentary — ideal body weight (lbs) × 15
active — ideal body weight (lbs) × 20
growing child — ideal body weight (lbs) × 20
4. Distribute calories during day to match insulin effects, e.g.: 2/7 at each of 3 meals plus 1/7 at bedtime.
5. Reduce proportion of fat to 20% of calories; increase carbohydrate to 60% of calories.
6. Fat should have a reduced proportion from animal sources and more from fish and vegetable sources (i.e. lowered amount of saturated lipids and cholesterol). Measure plasma lipids before and after initial 4 weeks.
7. Carbohydrates should be complex starches (as in bread, rice, potato, pasta and other cereal products). Rapidly absorbed simple sugars and oligosaccharides are reserved for hypoglycaemic episodes only and have no place in the usual diet.

8. Some fibres (non-absorbable carbohydrates) such as guar gum,
   pectins and those in pulses (peas and beans) reduce insulin
   requirements when mixed with other foods — probably by slowing
   and lowering glucose absorption curve. A high fibre diet should be
   encouraged, but fibre in the form of leguminous seeds (e.g. soya
   beans) more than cereals is beneficial in diabetic control.

ORAL HYPOGLYCAEMIC AGENTS (see Table 34)

Oral agents are used — particularly in adult onset diabetes without
ketosis — when an initial 4 week trial on diet alone has failed to
control symptoms and hyperglycaemia.

1. **Sulphonylureas**
   a. Stimulate insulin release from pancreatic β-cells. Also hepatic
      and peripheral hypoglycaemic actions. Possibly increase insulin
      receptor density. Functioning pancreatic tissue necessary for
      action.
   b. Increased appetite and weight gain.
   c. Can produce hypoglycaemia.
   d. Other toxicity: rashes, blood dyscrasias, flushing with alcohol
      (chlorpropamide), hyponatraemia. Contraindicated in liver
      failure.
   e. Hypoglycaemia potentiated by clofibrate, phenylbutazone,
      monoamine oxidase inhibitors.
   f. Hypoglycaemia reduced by steroids, thiazides, frusemide, the
      Pill, thyroxin, nicotinic acid.

2. **Biguanide (metformin)**
   a. Reduced glucose production by the liver.
   b. Reduced appetite and hence aids weight loss. Also metallic
      taste, vomiting, diarrhoea. Reduces absorption of folic acid and
      vitamin B_{12}.
   c. Lactic acidosis — uncommon but 60% mortality.

Special problems in diabetes

1. *Infections*
   a. Even minor viral infections may raise insulin needs 30%.
   b. Dose of insulin must be promptly reduced after infection.
   c. Patients often stop insulin if vomiting and not eating.
   d. Use sliding scale based on blood and/or uring tests with 4
      hourly insulin.

2. *Surgery*
   a. Admit to hospital 48 hours before operation.
   b. Change (if not treated normally in this way) to three times daily
      soluble insulin.

Table 33 Management of hyperglycaemic coma (Guy's Hospital — from H Keen & J Jarrett)

1. History and examination — previous severity and treatment of diabetes and complications. Look for infection, infarction, trauma. Monitor ECG, temperature, pulse, respiration, blood pressure hourly.
2. Set up i.v. line and CVP line; take blood initially for glucose, electrolytes, arterial pH, PO_2 PCO_2, FBP and culture. Repeat blood glucose hourly. Na^+ and K^+ hourly for 2 hours then 4 hourly.
3. Nasogastric tube and aspirate stomach contents.
4. Catheterise bladder — test urine hourly: volume output, glucose, ketones.
5. Give the following:

Time (hrs)	Fluid (saline)	Potassium	Insulin		Bicarbonate
			i.m. or Continuous i.v. infusion (by pump or i.v. drip)		Only give if considerable acidosis:
			i.m.	i.v.	Arterial pH
0–1	1 l in first 30 mins then 0.5 l in second 30 mins.	13 mmol/h initially	5 U	5 U/h	<7 : 100 mmol HCO_3 with 26 mmol K^+
1–2	1 l/h	Change rate of administration of K according to plasma K:	5 U	5 U/h	7.0–7.1 : 50 mmol HCO_3 with 13 mmol K^+
2–3	0.5 l/h				∴ give over 30–40 mins.

Fluid (saline) additional note for first period:
(NaCl 154 mM; but change to 5% glucose when blood glucose <14 mmol/l; if blood Na^+ >155 mmol/l then give NaCl 77 mM)

Table 33 (continued)

Time (hrs)	Fluid (saline)	Potassium	Insulin	Bicarbonate
3–4	0.5 l/h	Plasma K (mmol/l): >6, 6–4.5, 4.5–3, <3	If no fall in blood glucose then switch to i.v. regime.	If no fall in blood glucose then double rate.
4–5	0.25 l/h	∴ Give K (mMol/h): 0, 13, 26, 39	When blood glucose <14 mmol/l switch to 4-hourly s.c. injections according to urine glucose:	Measure pH 30 mins after and repeat schedule until pH<7.1.
5–6	0.25 l/h		Urine glucose: 2%, 1%, <1% — ∴ give insulin s.c. 4-hourly: 32 U, 16 U, 8 U	

Table 34 Oral hypoglycaemic agents

Drug	Metabolism and elimination	T½ (h)	Duration of action (h)	Special features
1. SULPHONYLUREAS				
Tolbutamide	Oxidised in liver, excreted in urine	4–5	6–12	Alcohol enhances action and may produce mild disulfiram type reaction. Less active in chronic alcoholics
Chlorpropamide	Little metabolised, mainly excreted unchanged in urine	36	60	Responsible for half cases of sulphonylurea hypoglycaemia. Some individuals develop severe disulfiram effect with alcohol
Glibenclamide	95% metabolised to inactive hydroxylated derivatives Excreted in bile and urine	1.5–2.5	12–24	Mildly diuretic. Avoid in elderly. Contraindicated in renal failure
Glipizide	85% metabolised to inactive hydroxyl derivative	2.5–4	6–10	
2. BIGUANIDE				
Metformin	Entirely excreted by kidneys	3–6	3–6	Contraindicated in renal failure

   c. During surgery i.v. infusion of 3 U insulin/h plus 6 g glucose/h. Infusion rates may have to be modified to produce blood glucose levels of 6–8 mmol/l (monitor hourly).

   d. Continue c. until oral feeding with intermittent insulin injections can be resumed — initially the sliding scale is used.

   e. Patients with such mild diabetes that insulin is not required during operations should have monitoring of glucose levels into the postoperative period.

3. *Pregnancy*

   a. Increased risk to fetus and increased incidence of congenital malformations. Deterioration of established retinopathy and nephropathy in mother.

   b. Supervision essential from the earliest stages of pregnancy to

produce exemplary blood glucose control. Single dose insulin
regimes changed to multiple doses.
c. Renal threshold for glucose falls during pregnancy and therefore
urine testing is unsuitable. Change to blood testing with
Dextrostix. Modify insulin and meals accordingly.
d. Renal glycosuria can cause starvation ketosis. Do not increase
insulin dose but raise carbohydrate intake.
e. Any problem with control is treated immediately in hospital.
Check control with HbA_{1c} and with preprandial blood glucose
(should be <7.2 mmol/l).
f. Obstetrician and physician together see patient: 4 weekly up to
28 weeks, 2 weekly up to 36 weeks and weekly up to
delivery. Accurate assessment of fetal development needed to
choose time of delivery.

4. *Labour*
a. Induce on morning of chosen day. No breakfast but set up drip
of 10% glucose with 10 U soluble insulin/500 ml and infuse
100 ml/hr.
Alternatively: 10 g/h glucose by drip and 1–2 U insulin/h by
syringe pump.
b. Monitor blood glucose hourly and change rate of drip if
necessary.
c. After rupture of membranes, apply electrodes to fetal scalp
and monitor ECG. Measure fetal blood pH. Deliver rapidly if
bradycardia, tachycardia or pH falls below 7.2.
d. Paediatrician present at delivery. Increased risk of
hypoglycaemia, hypocalcaemia, hyperbilirubinaemia and
congenital malformations.

General care of diabetics
1. Maintain blood glucose in ideal range, avoiding preprandial
hyperglycaemia and post insulin hypoglycaemia.
2. Continuing education. British Diabetic Association very helpful
particularly with diabetes in childhood.
3. Many problems in children: increases in physical activity and
emotional crises can lead to hypoglycaemia; low renal threshold;
failure to empty bladder.
4. Stop smoking; treat hyperlipidaemia.
5. Regular symptom enquiry and examination of eyes, feet and urine.
6. Antihypertensive treatment (β-blockers or ACE inhibitors) improve
survival in patients with diabetic nephropathy.

THYROID GLAND
The thyroid hormones are thyroxine (T_4) and liothyronine (T_3).
    Excessive production of T_3 and T_4 produces thyrotoxicosis:
deficiency produces myxoedema or cretinism.

Secretion of T_3 and T_4 increased by TSH (released in response to low plasma levels of T_3 and T_4) and by immunoglobulins (thyroid stimulating and thyroid growth IgG) with TSH activity (not affected by T_3 and T_4 levels).

Actions of T_3 and T_4

Hormone action	*Clinical consequence in hyper- or hypothyroidism*
1. Stimulation of metabolism	Heat intolerance, increased appetite with weight loss, raised metabolic rate in hyperthyroidism; hypothermia and coma in myxoedema
2. Promotion of growth and development	Dwarfism and mental deficiency in cretinism
3. Sensitisation to sympathetic effects by increasing β receptors	Eyelid retraction, tachycardia, tremor, hyperactive reflexes in hyperthyroidism

Pharmacokinetics	*Thyroxine (T_4)*	*Liothyronine (T_3)*
Gut absorption	Complete	Complete
Latency before action starts	24 h	6 h
Peak effect	7–10 d	24 h
$T_{1/2}$	6–7 d	2 d or less
Metabolism	Conjugation and enterohepatic circulation 20% is converted to T_3 in tissues	Conjugation and enterohepatic circulation
Normal levels	50–10 µg/l (80% of circulating thyroid hormone) 99.95% bound to thyroid binding globulin	1–1.6 µg/l (20% of circulating thyroid hormone) 99.5% bound to plasma protein

Therefore, ratio of free T_4:T_3 is 4–5:1. Main secretion of gland is T_4 which acts as the prohormone for T_3.

Uses of T_3 and T_4

T_4 is standard treatment for hypothyroidism (adult, childhood and neonatal).
T_3 is used in the initial treatment of myxoedema coma and other severe hypothyroid states when a rapid response is needed.
T_4 may reduce the size of non-toxic goitres which have not responded to iodine alone.
T_4 used in Hashimoto's thyroiditis and in thyroid carcinoma.

Toxicity
Cardiac — tachycardia, angina, myocardial infarction, congestive
   failure, arrhythmias, sudden death.
Diarrhoea.
Tremor, restlessness, heat intolerance.

Treatment of hyperthyroidism

1. Medical
Children and young adults
Preparation for surgery
Mild — moderate disease
Thyroid gland not greatly enlarged
Elderly patients rendered euthyroid on drugs, can then be left
   indefinitely on a small maintenance dose.

2. Surgery
Large gland
Compression of neighbouring structures
Nodular gland, toxic adenoma.

3. Radioactive iodine (I^{131})
Postoperative recurrence
Surgery contraindicated
Failed drug therapy in an adult.

Medical management

1. Long-term treatment

	Drug	Toxicity
Block iodination of tyrosyl residues and reduce IgG production	{ Carbimazole { Propylthiouracil	Itching and rashes can be treated with antihistamines without stopping the drug. Agranulocytosis is often preceded by a sore throat (stop drug). Over-treatment causes hypothyroidism

   Drugs usually given for 1½–2 years then slowly withdrawn. 50%
relapse when drugs stopped and require continued treatment.
Euthyroid state is usually attained within 4–6 weeks of treatment; the
dose is then reduced and continued for 18 months. Carbimazole with
thyroxine (blocking-replacement) is an alternative regimen and is
usually given for 18 months. Propranolol is added to antithyroid drugs
to produce a rapid relief from toxic symptoms and to control tremor
and supraventricular tachyarrhythmias.

2. Short term management
Preparation for surgery
Treating severe disease until I^{131} starts to become effective
   a. Start antithyroid drug.
   b. Add propranolol — reduces restlessness, tremor, sweating, anxiety. β-blockers act by:
      (i) reducing peripheral sympathetic activity
      (ii) blocking formation of T_3 from T_4.
   c 7–10 days before surgery, iodine (0.5 ml Lugol's aqueous iodine solution 8 hourly) is given. This is a powerful but short-lived inhibitor of hormone release which also reduces the vascularity of the gland.

3. Pregnancy
   a. Operate if severe disease or large goitre in early or mid-pregnancy.
   b. Antithyroid drugs can be given throughout pregnancy if surgery is not undertaken, but thyroxine is not added.
   c. Radioactive iodine is contraindicated.

4. Thyroid crisis
   a. Via intravenous line give fluids, propranolol and hydrocortisone succinate.
   and
   b. Via nasogastric tube give iodine solution and carbimazole.

5. Eye signs
   a. Usually resolve with treatment but 5% guanethidine eye drops may improve appearance.
   b. Visual failure — prednisolone 60 mg daily with surgical decompression if unsuccessful.

OSTEOPOROSIS

No known measure reverses osteoporosis.
Treatment aims to maintain current skeletal integrity and prevent further loss.
1. Patient education: stress the importance of exercise.
2. Avoid immobilisation and prolonged confinement to bed.
3. Diet should contain adequate protein, minerals and vitamins. Calcium intake should be adequate (over 750 mg daily). Vitamin D (1000 U calciferol/day) or its metabolites should not be given in absence of deficiency or osteomalacia. Supplementary calcium 1.5–2 g/day is not of value.
4. Oestrogens are of proven benefit if started shortly after menopause. Possible risk of endometrial cancer reduced by adding cyclical progestogen.

5. Anabolic steroids, e.g. stanozolol — helpful in males with Klinefelter's syndrome and hypogonadal states, but not clinically useful in postmenopausal osteoporosis.
6. Other measures:
   Fluoride stimulates osteoblasts and increases trabecular bone mass in patients with severe osteoporosis.
   Calcitonin (injected or intranasal) inhibits bone resorption.
   Diphosphonates such as etidronate are possibly of benefit in steroid-induced osteoporosis.

OSTEOMALACIA

Vitamin D is a group of substances which can cure rickets and other forms of dietary osteomalacia. It includes:
   ergocalciferol (calciferol; vitamin D_2)
   cholecalciferol (vitamin D_3)
   alfacalcidol (1α-hydroxycholecalciferol)
   calcitriol (1,25 dihydroxycholecalciferol)
   Dietary deficiency is treated with oral calciferol in small doses (10 μg daily). When the deficiency is due to chronic liver disease or malabsorption, larger doses (1 mg) are needed.

RENAL BONE DISEASE

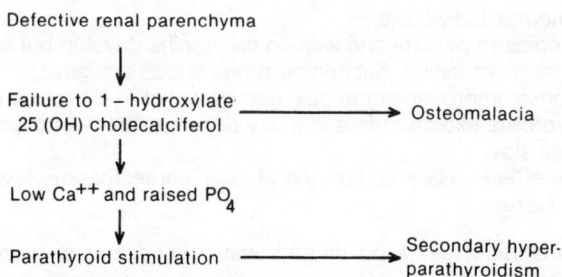

Defective renal parenchyma

↓

Failure to 1 – hydroxylate ⟶ Osteomalacia
25 (OH) cholecalciferol

↓

Low Ca^{++} and raised PO_4

↓

Parathyroid stimulation ⟶ Secondary hyperparathyroidism

Fig. 16.2

1. Osteomalacia or hyperparathyroidism: give calcitriol or alfacalcidol, but avoid hypercalcaemia.
2. Hypocalcaemia also treated by oral calcium and phosphate binding agents (e.g. aluminium hydroxide). Reduction of phosphate may reduce secondary hyperparathyroidism.

TREATMENT OF HYPOPARATHYROIDISM

1. High dose calciferol (5 mg daily) or dihydrotachysterol.

2. Essential: regular follow-up (initially, weekly) to check plasma calcium concentration.

PAGET'S DISEASE OF BONE

Most patients are asymptomatic and require no treatment. Indications for treatment are:
1. Bone pain unresponsive to simple analgesics.
2. Hypercalcaemia due to immobilisation.
3. Nerve root or cord compression — paraplegia may be reversed but deafness rarely improves.
4. Juvenile Paget's disease — only some types respond.
5. Reduction of high cardiac output failure (rare).

Progression of disease, especially in young patients, may be prevented (unproven). No improvement in rate of fracture healing with treatment.

Treatment monitored by symptomatic response, alkaline phosphatase, urinary hydroxyproline excretion. Additional methods — X-rays, bone scans, skin temperature, radio-calcium kinetics.

Two main treatments:

1. Calcitonins (pork calcitonin and salcatonin)
Inhibit osteoclast activity so reducing bone resorption. Degree of hypocalcaemia produced related to prevailing bone resorption rate so produces greater fall in children, thyrotoxicosis and Paget's disease than in normal individuals.

Antibodies to porcine and salmon calcitonins develop but rarely cause treatment failure. Salmon hormone is less antigenic.

Response: improvement in pain occurs within 1–2 weeks. Urinary hydroxyproline excretion falls in a day or two, alkaline phosphatase falls more slowly.

Adverse effects. Nausea, flushing of face, paraesthesiae, fever, metallic taste.

2. Biphosphonates (disodium etidronate, disodium pamidronate and sodium clodronate).

Pharmacology
Inhibit growth and dissolution of hydroxyapalite crystals; reduce bone absorption and turnover.

Adverse effects
GI intolerance, especially with higher dose. May cause hypocalcaemia.

HYPERCALCAEMIA

Establish cause. Remove calcium from diet. Rehydrate. A loop diuretic may be added to intravenous sodium chloride 0.9%. In some patients,

drugs may be needed:
  binders of alimentary calcium, e.g. sodium cellulose phosphate
  rapid, short action — plicamycin
  slower action — steroids, calcitonins
  intravenous chelating agents — trisodium edetate
  in malignancy — etidronate, pamidronate or clodronate.

17. Anti-infective chemotherapy

ANTIBACTERIAL DRUGS

Antibiotics
Compounds synthesised by microorganisms which kill or inhibit the growth of cells which produce disease (mainly microorganisms and neoplasms).

Chemotherapeutic substances
All compounds (synthetic and produced by living cells) which kill or inhibit the growth of cells which produce disease in the body.

Bactericidal
i.e. kills bacteria (e.g. penicillins, aminoglycosides).

Bacteriostatic
i.e. stops bacterial division: bacteria eliminated by host defences (e.g. tetracyclines, erythromycin).
NB Bactericidal/static distinction of little importance under most conditions in practice. However, bactericidal drugs should be used when phagocytic cells cannot get to site of infection (e.g. endocarditis) or in leucopenia. Giving bacteriostatic and cidal drugs together may be synergistic, additive or antagonistic, but usually no measurable disadvantage occurs.

SULPHONAMIDES

Use has greatly declined in recent years. Occasionally used for urinary infections and prophylaxis of meningococcal infection. However pyrimethamine with sulphadiazine is the treatment of choice for toxoplasmosis and co-trimoxazole in high doses is used to treat pneumocystis pneumonia. Silver sulphadiazine is applied to infected skin lesions, including burns.

Action
Block bacterial folic acid synthesis by combining with pteridine to form an inactive complex. This metabolic step is absent in man.

Toxicity
Rashes are common (including Stevens-Johnson syndrome).
Drug fever, dizziness, headache, malaise, crystalluria (especially with
sulphadiazine). Can produce anuria.
Acute renal toxicity can also occur due to intrarenal damage.
Kernicterus (when given in last 2 weeks of pregnancy or to a neonate)
because of displacement of unconjugated bilirubin from plasma
protein binding.
Haemolytic anaemia in G6PD deficiency.
Agranulocytosis, aplastic anaemia.

CO-TRIMOXAZOLE

This is a mixture of trimethoprim and sulphamethoxazole. It has been
used for urinary and respiratory tract infections, but because of
common allergy to the sulphonamide component, trimethoprim alone
is preferred.
   High dose co-trimoxazole is an agent of choice in treating
pneumonia due to *Pneumocystis carinii*.

TRIMETHOPRIM

Action
Competitive inhibitor of dihydrofolate reductase with affinity for
bacterial enzyme 50 000 times that for human. Thus inhibits
formation of 'active' folate.
   Potent broad-spectrum bacteriostatic agent. Resistance due to
resistant dihydrofolate reductase is increasing.

Toxicity
Nausea, vomiting, diarrhoea; rash; folate deficiency anaemia (only in
those with initially low folate stores). Possible teratogenic risk.

Use
For treatment and prophylaxis of urinary tract infections, respiratory
infections, prostatitis and invasive salmonella infections.
Contraindicated in pregnancy (because it is a folate antagonist).

β-LACTAM ANTIBIOTICS

These share a β-lactam ring in their molecular structure. They act by
interfering with synthesis of the bacterial cell wall. The group consists
of the penicillins, cephalosporins, cephamycins, monobactams and
carbapenems.

THE PENICILLINS

The penicillins are bactericidal. They diffuse well into body tissues and fluids (including the eye and fetus) but penetrate poorly into the CNS unless the meninges are inflamed.

In general penicillins have $T_{1/2}$ 1–2 h and are mainly eliminated in the urine (tubular secretion is blocked by probenecid).

Organisms sensitive to benzyl penicillin

G + ve cocci:
Staph aureus — not β-lactamase (penicillinase) producing strains
Strep. pneumoniae
β-haemolytic streptococci (Lancefield group A *Strep. pyogenes*)
Strep. viridans
G – ve cocci:
Neisseria gonorrhoeae
Neisseria meningitidis
G + ve bacilli:
Bacillus anthracis
Corynebacterium diphtheriae
Listeria monocytogenes
Clostridium sp. (and many other anaerobes except *Bacteroides fragilis*)
Spirochaetes:
Treponema pallidum
Treponema pertenue
Leptospira icterohaemorrhagiae
Actinomyces

Resistant organisms

Strep. faecalis
Neisseria gonorrhoeae (some strains)
Haemophilus influenzae
Penicillinase-producing staphylococci
Escherichia coli
Klebsiella
Proteus mirabilis
Serratia
Pseudomonas aeruginosa
Bacteroides fragilis

Penicillin toxicity

1. Hypersensitivity
Type 1 reactions (early):
  a. rash (common) — urticaria, erythema.
  b. anaphylaxis (rare) — circulatory collapse, bronchospasm, laryngeal oedema.
Serum sickness (type III reactions) — delayed by 2–12 days: fever, malaise, arthralgia, angioedema, erythema nodosum, exfoliative dermatitis, erythema multiforme, Stevens-Johnson syndrome.

2. *Neurotoxicity*
   a. only high doses (those which may be used with carbenicillin)
   b. anuria
   c. intrathecal injection of over 50 000 U
Encephalopathy can present as:
   fits, coma
   permanent sequelae
   death.

Table 35 Penicillins I

Drugs	Special features	Main uses
Benzylpenicillin	Highly active against susceptible organisms but destroyed by penicillinase. Does not penetrate well into the CSF. Injected	1. Serious infections needing parenteral antibiotic, e.g. meningitis, endocarditis, septicaemia. 2. Infections due to susceptible organisms, e.g. pneumococcal pneumonia, streptococcal pharyngitis, gonorrhoea, syphilis, soft tissue infections due to streptococci pyogenes and microaerophilic streptococci.
Ampicillin	*High concentrations in urine and bile.* Broad spectrum. Oral (can also be injected)	Urinary infections, acute exacerbations of chronic bronchitis, cholecystitis, Infections due to *H. influenzae (e.g. meningitis, arthritis, otitis media).*
Amoxycillin	*Better (× 2) intestinal absorption than ampicillin and higher tissue levels.* Otherwise same as ampicillin but possibly more active against *Strep. faecalis* and *Salmonella*. Oral (can also be injected)	As with ampicillin. Also *large single dose (3 g) before dental and other instrumental* procedures, in particular with valvular heart disease as SABE prophylaxis. *Also 2 × 3 g doses in acute urinary infections.* May penetrate *sputum* better than ampicillin. *Typhoid (as good as chloramphenicol).*

Talampicillin and pivampicillin are prodrugs of ampicillin

3. *Potassium and sodium overload because of salts in injectable forms*
4. *Ampicillin, amoxycillin, talampicillin* and *pivampicillin* produce rash (usually morbilliform) in about 8% of patients, more commonly in young women. A very high incidence of this reaction occurs in infectious mononucleosis and chronic lymphatic leukaemia.
5. *Diarrhoea with oral forms*

Table 36 Penicillins II — Active against β-lactamase producing bacteria

Drug	Special features	Main uses
1. *Inherent resistance to β-lactamase*		
Flucloxacillin	Well absorbed orally. Oral (or injected)	Infections due to β-lactamase producing Staph. is sole indication.
Temocillin	Injected	β-lactamase producing G negative bacteria (not pseudomonas)
2. *β-lactamase inhibition*		
Clavulanic acid has little intrinsic antibacterial activity but inhibits β-lactamase		
Amoxycillin + Clavulanate (Co-amoxiclav)	Activity against most amoxycillin- resistant *Staph. aureus, H. influenzae, Kl. aerogenes, E. coli* and Bacteroides sp. Oral	When sensitivity of amoxycillin-resistant organism demonstrated.
Ticarcillin + Clavulanate	Injected	Pseudomonas and proteus.

CEPHALOSPORINS AND CEPHAMYCINS (See Tables 39, 40, 41)

Inhibit bacterial cell wall synthesis by inhibiting transpeptidase formation of cross links in mucopeptide (as does penicillin).

Board spectrum agents although individual agents have enhanced activity against some pathogens. Not active against enterococci and Listeria

Toxicity
Hypersensitivity (10% penicillin sensitive patients cross-react). Haemorrhage is caused by some cephalosporins, especially latamoxef.

Cephamycins
Cefoxitin is active against *Bacteroides fragilis* and may be effective in treating abdominal sepsis.

OTHER β LACTAMS

1. Monobactam: **aztreonam** has a spectrum limited to Gram – ve aerobic bacteria including Pseudomonas, meningococcus and Haemophilus.
2. Carbapenem: **imipenem** has a very broad spectrum including Gram + ve and – ve bacteria. It is partially inactivated enzymically by the kidney but cilastin prevents this. It is neurotoxic in high doses.

Table 37 Penicillins III — Active against *Pseudomonas aeruginosa*
1. Despite broad spectra solely used for suspected or proven Pseudomonas (or occasionally ampicillin-resistant Proteus) infections
2. All hydrolysed by β-lactamases so 90% *Staph. aureus* and 40% *E. coli* resistant
3. Synergistic with aminoglycosides (but should not be put in same container together)
4. All given i.v.

Drug	Special features	Main uses
1. *Carbenicillin and related drugs*		
Carbenicillin	Neurotoxicity NB: 30 g carbenicillin contains 163 mM Na$^+$ so danger of overload	Has been replaced by ticarcillin
Ticarcillin	Twice as active as carbenicillin 20 g contains 107 mM Na$^+$. Used with clavulanic acid against β-lactamase-producing bacteria	Severe infections due to Pseudomonas and Proteus
2. *Ureidopenicillins*		
Azlocillin and piperacillin	More active then ticarcillin	Severe Pseudomonas infections. Used with aminoglycosides for Pseudomonas septicaemia

Table 38 Mecillinams

Drug	Administration	Special features	Main uses
Mecillinam	Parenteral administration only	An imidinopenicillin chemically related to penicillins but with different action on bacterial cell wall. Destroyed by some but not all penicillinases. Not absorbed from gut. Excreted in urine	Active against G – ve bacilli, but excluding *Ps. aeruginosa*. Used for severe G – ve infections with enteric bacteria
Pivmecillinam	Oral	Pivaloyloxymethyl ester, a prodrug of mecillinam. Absorbed from gut and hydrolysed to free mecillinam	Urinary infections and salmonellosis

ERYTHROMYCIN

A macrolide.

Spectrum similar but not identical to benzylpenicillin so useful for patients allergic to penicillin.

Pharmacology

Bacteriostatic. Binds to bacterial but not human ribosome 50S subunit to inhibit protein synthesis.

Erythromycin base destroyed by acid so given as enteric coated tablets or as esters (succinate or estolate) which are less susceptible and better absorbed. Base and stearate are poorly absorbed if given with food.

No need for dose adjustment in renal failure.

Serious toxicity unusual but nausea common with oral drug.

Cholestatic jaundice with eosinophilia can arise after 14 days' treatment.

Table 39 Cephalosporins — First generation
1. Rarely agents of first choice: becoming obsolete.
2. All hydrolysed by β-lactamases.

Drug	Administration	Toxicity	Uses
Cephazolin	Injected	Allergic rashes	No absolute
Cephradine	Oral or injected	Nausea	indications but are
		Diarrhoea and colitis	used for sensitive G
		Fever	+ ve and G – ve
		Arthralgia	infections.
		Dizziness	Oral agents used for
			urinary infections
Cephalexin	Oral		
Cephradine	Oral		
Cefadroxil	Oral		

Table 40 Cephalosporins — Second Generation

Drug	Administration	Special features	Uses
Cefuroxime	Injected	Relatively resistant to β-lactamase	Similar range to 1st generation but greater activity against *H. influenzae* and *N. gonorrhoeae*
Cefamandole	Injected		
Cefaclor	Oral		Urinary infections

Table 41 Cephalosporins — Third generation
Variable stability to β-lactamase
Variable activity against *Pseudomonas aeruginosa*, inactive against *Strep. faecalis*

Drug	Administration	Special features	Uses
Cefotaxime and ceftizoxime	Injected	Active against entero bacteria, but little action against G + ve bacteria	Specific G – ve infections
Cefsoludin	Injected	Narrow spectrum	Specifically for Pseudomonas
Ceftazidime	Injected	Active against many G – ve bacteria	Pseudomonas and other G – ve infections
Cefixime	Oral	Can cause diarrhoea and pseudomembranous colitis	G + ve and G – ve infections but not staphylococci or anaerobes

Uses
Penicillin sensitive patients, e.g. for strep., staph. and pneumococcal infections, prophylaxis bacterial endocarditis, syphilis.
Legionnaires' disease.
Campylobacter enteritis.
Chlamydial pneumonia in infants.
Chlamydial infection in pregnancy (tetracycline would harm fetus).
Mycoplasma pneumonia in infants (tetracycline used in adults).

Clarithromycin is a macrolide derived from erythromycin which has greater activity and higher tissue penetration than the parent drug.
Reduce dose in renal failure.

AMINOGLYCOSIDES

Common properties:
1. Inhibit bacterial ribosomal protein synthesis.
2. Spectrum includes aerobic and facultatively anaerobic Gram – ve bacilli and cocci and staphylococci but streptococci and other Gram + ves and strict anaerobes are resistant.
3. Three main types of acquired resistance:
   a. ribosome level (streptomycin only)
   b. decreased transport of antibiotic into bacterium — may affect several aminoglycosides
   c. plasmid transmitted enzymes which adenylate, phosphorylate or acetylate antibiotic.
4. Often synergistic with β-lactam antibiotics.
5. Very little absorbed p.o. so given parenterally or topically.

6. Narrow therapeutic range — ototoxic and nephrotoxic. Not given with potentially ototoxic drugs such as frusemide. Also neuromuscular blockade and contraindicated in myasthenia.
7. Plasma $T_{1/2}$ about 2 h. Monitoring of levels important for safe parenteral use.
8. Renal excretion so caution in renal failure.
9. Avoid in pregnancy — cross placenta to cause 8th cranial nerve damage.

TETRACYCLINES

These act preferentially on bacterial ribosomes but also have some anti anabolic action on mammalian cells (and thus worsen uraemia). The tetracyclines are broad spectrum and are the treatment of choice

Table 42 Aminoglycosides

Drug	Toxicity	Comments
Gentamicin	Vestibular damage. Reversible nephrotoxicity	Broad spectrum with activity against Pseudomonas. Used for 'blind' treatment of serious infections. Usually given with a penicillin or metronidazole
Tobramycin	Vestibular damage. Less nephrotoxic than gentamicin	More active than gentamicin against Pseudomonas but less active for other bacteria
Amikacin	Mainly high-tone deafness	Potentially widest spectrum as stable to 8 of the 9 bacterial aminoglycoside-inactivating enzymes. Used for gentamicin resistant organisms
Kanamycin	Deafness mainly but mild nephrotoxicity relatively common	Superseded by gentamicin
Neomycin	Sensitisation if used topically. Prolonged oral administration may produce malabsorption syndrome. Not used systemically because of deafness	Topical for Staphylococcal and Gram-negative infections. Gut sterilisation in liver disease
Netilmicin	Less ototoxic than gentamicin	Less active than gentamicin against pseudomonas but more active against other G – ve bacilli
Streptomycin	Ototoxic. Contact dermatitis	Reserved for TB, otherwise superceded by other aminoglycosides

Table 43 Antibacterial agents with special uses

Drug	Toxicity	Uses
Sodium fusidate	Low toxicity: mild GT disturbances. Allergy. Reversible changes in liver function tests and occasionally jaundice	Narrow spectrum; reserved for penicillin- resistant staphylococci
Glycopeptides:		
Vancomycin	Can only be given intravenously — necrosis if extravasates. Thrombophlebitis. Renal damage. Rash including 'red man syndrome'	Use-restricted to serious refractory G +ve infections, e.g. Staphylococci, Streptococci and pseudomembranous colitis
Teicoplanin	Nausea, anaphylaxis, leucopenia	Similar uses to vancomycin, but can be given i.m. as well as i.v.
Chloramphenicol	Reversible, dose-dependent inhibition of erythropoiesis. Also irreversible idiosyncratic marrow aplasia (1 : 30,000). Grey syndrome in neonates	Reserved for life-threatening infections including typhoid and Haemophilus meningitis (good penetration into meninges and brain).

for infections by chlamydia, rickettsiae, mycoplasma and Lyme disease. They are also used for chronic bronchitis, acne and rosacea. Minocycline has a broader spectrum and has been used for prophylaxis against meningococcal meningitis.

When given to children under the age of 12 years and to pregnant women, they cause discolouration of the teeth.

Tetracycline, chlortetracycline, oxytetracycline, demeclocycline and lymecycline are contraindicated in chronic renal disease. However doxycycline and minocycline do not worsen renal failure and can be used in kidney disease.

Doxycycline and minocycline absorption is not decreased by salts of calcium, iron and magnesium, whereas the absorption of other tetracyclines is inibited by foods and drugs containing these salts.

QUINOLONES

These act by inhibition of bacterial DNA gyrase which controls DNA supercoiling.

Nalidixic acid, norfloxacin and cinoxacin are quinolones used for uncomplicated urinary infections. Other fluoroquinones include ciprofloxacin, enoxacin, and ofloxacin. These all have a broad spectrum of activity.

Table 44 Drugs for anaerobic and other infections

Drug	Pharmacokinetics	Toxicity	Clinical use
Metronidazole (Tinidazole is similar but has a longer action)	Well absorbed from gut and across mucosae. $T_{1/2} = 6-10$ h. Penetrates into abscesses, bone, CNS and milk. Excreted in saliva and urine. Undergoes extensive hepatic metabolism so reduce dose in hepatic failure	CNS: Reversible peripheral neuropathy (1–3%), ataxia, vertigo, headaches, fits. GI: (5–10%) nausea, vomiting, metallic taste, diarrhoea. Others: fever, reversible neutropenia. Interactions: Disulfiram-like with ethanol; potentiates warfarin and coumarins	Anaerobic infections. *Trichomonas vaginalis*. Acute ulcerative gingivitis. *Giardia lamblia* infections. Acute amoebic dysentery, hepatitis and abscess. Tropical ulcer, dracontiasis, *Dracunculus medinensis* infestations. Crohn's disease
Clindamycin (Lincomycin similar, but less well absorbed)	Well absorbed from gut. $T_{1/2} = 2$ h. 85% undergoes hepatic metabolism and $T_{1/2}$ increased by cirrhosis, hepatitis or old age. Concentrated in bile and macrophages and polymorphs (so enters abscesses) but poor penetration into CNS. Levels in bone about 40% plasma level	GI: diarrhoea (10–20%) — dose-related due to toxic effect on mucosa. Also more serious pseudomembranous colitis (2%). Allergy: Rash (3–5%) eosinophilia	Anaerobic infections, including Bacteroides. Effective also in staphylococcal and pneumococcal infections. Used in staphylococcal bone and joint infections and abdominal sepsis

Ciprofloxacin is effective orally and penetrates into cells, lung and prostate. Activity is present against G +ve and G –ve bacteria, but is not effective against bacteroides and pneumococcus. It is most useful against G –ve infections. Plasma levels of theophylline are raised.

Acrosoxacin is used only for the treatment of gonorrhoea in patients allergic to penicillin.

PROPHYLAXIS OF INFECTIVE ENDOCARDITIS

Required by patients with
1. Rheumatic and 'degenerative' valvular disease.
2. Congenital heart disease.
3. Prosthetic heart valves.

For the following procedures
1. Dental, e.g. extractions, scaling.
2. Genito-urinary, e.g. instrumentation, complicated vaginal delivery.
3. Gastrointestinal endoscopy and surgery.
4. Cardiac surgery.

Principles
1. Bactericidal antibiotics required.
2. Administration immediately prior to procedure — prevents bacterial antibiotic resistance.
3. Effective antibiotic levels maintained for at least 10 hours after procedure.

Methods
Oral amoxycillin — 3 g 1 h before procedure
If allergic to penicillin
Oral erythromycin 1.5 g of stearate 1–2 h before procedure then 500 mg 6 h later.
Or
Oral clindamycin 600 mg 1 h before procedure.

TREATMENT OF TUBERCULOSIS

General principles
1. At least 3 drugs given during initial phase and 2 drugs during continuation phase to prevent emergence of resistance.
2. Combination includes one first line bactericidal drug.
3. Poor compliance is commonest cause of failure, so drugs often given in combined formulations.
4. Tubercle bacillus grows slowly so treatment lasts months.

Standard regimen
For 6 months: isoniazid plus rifampicin, with the first 2 months supplemented with pyrazinamide. Ethambutol and streptomycin are

Table 45 Drug used solely for urinary infections

Drug	Pharmacokinetics	Toxicity	Uses
Nitrofurantoin	Absorbed well by mouth. 1/3 excreted unchanged in urine (100 μg/ml urine attained on usual oral dose — but low concentrations in plasma) $T\frac{1}{2} = 1$ h	Nausea common. Peripheral neuropathy if blood levels high, thus contraindicated by renal failure. Hypersensitivity (5%), produces rashes, fever and hepatitis (with + ve ANF). Rarely: bone marrow depression; pulmonary infiltration; Haemolytic anaemia if G6PD deficient	Gram-negative urinary pathogens: E. coli MIC for Klebsiella spp. <35 μg/ml (Proteus spp. usually resistant; Pseudomonas always resistant)
Nalidixic acid	Absorbed well by mouth. Concentrated in urine above blood levels. Dose not accumulate in moderate renal failure but toxic cumulation in severe renal disease	Toxicity uncommon; GI disturbances; rashes; visual disturbances; raised intracranial pressure and fits. Haemolytic anaemia if G6PD deficient	Gram-negative organisms MIC 10 μg/ml (apart from Pseudomonas and Bacteroides spp.)
Cinoxacin	Rapidly absorbed by mouth. 60% excreted unchanged in urine. $T\frac{1}{2} = 1-1\frac{1}{2}$ h	Toxicity increased in renal failure. GI disturbances. Hypersensitivity (urticaria; rashes; oedema). Transient changes in liver function tests. Not known if safe in pregnancy	Similar spectrum to nalidixic acid. Used in acute and chronic urinary tract infections

Table 46 First line anti-tuberculous drugs

Drug	Pharmacology	Pharmacokinetics	Adverse effects
Isoniazid	Bactericidal. Interferes with mycolic acid synthesis in bacterial cell wall. Active against intracellular organisms	Well absorbed with high CSF levels. Mainly hepatic elimination by genetically determined acetylation (see page 33) $T_{1/2} < 80$ min fast, >140 min slow. Inhibits phenytoin and warfarin metabolism	Peripheral neuropathy (mainly slow acetylators) — prevented by pyridoxine 10 mg/day. Disturbance of hepatic function — rarely hepatocellular failure, usually in old or alcoholics (? mainly fast acetylators). Occasionally fever, rash, lymphadenopathy, convulsions, psychosis
Rifampicin	Bactericidal. Inhibits bacterial DNA dependent RNA polymerase	Well absorbed with high CSF levels. Deacetylated by liver and excreted in bile. $T_{1/2} = 1\frac{1}{2} - 5$ h. Enzyme induction causes interactions with pill, anticoagulants, etc	Transient elevation of hepatic enzymes — serious hepatotoxicity uncommon (mainly in alcoholics or in pre-existing liver disease). 'Flu' syndrome after high doses. Colours urine, tears, sweat, sputum red
Ethambutol	Bacteriostatic	Well absorbed but CSF poorly penetrated. Mainly eliminated unchanged in urine. $T_{1/2} = 5 - 6$ h.	Retrobulbar neuritis, 1% on high doses (usually reversible) — important to test vision. Polyneuritis. Pruritus
Pyrazinamide	Bactericidal	Well absorbed with high CSF levels — used for TB meningitis	Hepatotoxicity with occasional acute necrosis. Nausea and vomiting. Arthralgia, hyperuricaemia and gout.

(Streptomycin also used)

Table 47 Second line anti-tuberculous drugs

Drug	Special features and usefulness	Toxicity
Prothionamide*	Rarely used because of GI toxicity	Gastric irritation Liver damage Neuropathy Mental disturbance
Thiacetazone	Cheap, but use limited because of toxicity	High incidence of rashes
Cycloserine	Main use in resistance to more conventional drugs. The most toxic of the second line drugs	Mental disturbance Fits
Capreomycin	Similar to streptomycin in actions and toxicity — but may be useful in patients with hypersensitivity or for resistant organisms	Ototoxicity ⎫ with high Nephrotoxicity ⎭ plasma levels Hypokalaemia Hypocalcaemia Hypomagnesaemia
PAS	Largely abandoned because of low efficacy and high toxicity. $T_{1/2} = 1$ h	Gastric irritation Hepatitis Rashes (5–10% of patients)

*Ethionamide is similar

included if resistance is suspected. Chemotherapy is prolonged for a further 3–6 months (9–12 months in all) in tuberculous meningitis and in some forms of lymphadenopathy and in bone and joint tuberculosis.

LEPROSY

Mainstay was dapsone but resistance increasing and rifampicin and clofazimine also used, with dapsone.

In paucibacillary disease dapsone daily and rifampicin monthly are given for 6 months.

In multibacillary disease, clofazimine is given with dapsone and rifampicin for at least 2 years up to smear negativity.

ANTIMALARIALS

1. Prophylaxis

It is recommended that drugs are started one week before travel into an endemic area and continued (apart from mefloquine) for 4 weeks after leaving. Prophylaxis does not give total protection, and thus nets and repellants are very important.

Children and pregnant women should (ideally) not travel to endemic areas.

Drugs used to prevent malaria:
  a. *4-amino quinolines*:
    Chloroquine 300 mg weekly. Not usually toxic at this dose, but prolonged treatment can cause retinopathy.

b. *Folate reductase inhibitors*:
   Proguanil 200 mg daily. Can exacerbate folate deficiency.
c. *Chloroquine-resistant falciparum malaria*:
   (i) maloprim (pyrimethamine 12.5 mg with dapsone 100 mg) weekly.
   (ii) fansidar (pyrimethamine 25 mg with sulphadoxine 0.5 g) weekly. Can cause serious skin reactions
   (iii) mefloquine for short term (<3 weeks) travel.

2. Treatment of acute attack
a. Chloroquine
In vivax terminates acute attack but not radically curative.
In falciparum usually curative but most is now resistant and quinine or mefloquine is therefore used.
Total oral dose 1.5 g (or 30 mg/kg):
   600 mg intially
   300 mg after 6 h
   300 mg daily for 2 days.
In severe falciparum:
   5–10 mg/kg i.v. every 12–24 h (each dose given over 4 h).
Toxicity in these doses:
   headache, visual disturbances
   pruritus
   GI disturbances.

	Chloroquine	Quinine
Absorption	Almost completely absorbed from intestine. Can be given i.v. and i.m. Excretion accelerated by acidifying urine. High concentration in all tissues.	Complete absorption from intestine. Peak levels at 1.3 h. Irritant and poor absorption i.m. and s.c.
$T_{1/2}$	120 h	10 h (but prolonged in falciparum m.)
Elimination	50–70% renal excretion unchanged, some hepatic metabolism.	95% metabolised in liver.
Non-malarial uses	Rheumatoid arthritis; Discoid lupus; Possible benefit in SLE; Photoallergic reactions; *Clonorchis sinensis, Fasciola hepatica,* and *Paragonimus* infestations	Myotonia congenita 0.3–0.6 g 8-hourly Dystrophia myotonica 0.3–0.6 g 8-hourly Nocturnal leg cramps 0.2–3 g at night.

	Chloroquine	Quinine
Toxicity	Prolonged treatment with large doses: retinopathy with loss of central acuity, macular pigmentation, retinal artery constriction. Lichenoid skin eruptions, bleaching of hair. Reduced T waves on ECG. Weight loss. Ototoxicity.	Large doses: cinchonism — tinnitus, deafness, headache, nausea, visual disturbances. GI disturbances. Rashes, fever, delirium, tremor, fits, coma, renal failure, haemolytic anaemia, purpura.

b. Quinine
Mainly used to treat an acute attack of chloroquine-resistant falciparum.

Usual oral treatment: 600 mg every 8 h for 7 days followed by 3 tablets of Fansidar (pyrimethamine 75 mg with sulphadoxine 1.5 g) to ensure eradication of disease. For recrudescence of treated malaria or for severe falciparum by i.v. infusion (20 mg/kg over 4 h, then after 8–12 h, 10 mg/kg over 4 h every 8–12 h).

c. Mefloquine
Used as an alternative to quinine in the treatment of chloroquine-resistant falciparum. 50% of patients develop GI disturbances, dizziness, nausea, weakness.

3. Treatment of relapse
Not usually required with *P. falciparum* and *P. malariae*. Following treatment of acute attack of *P. vivax*, prevent or treat febrile episodes with primaquine 15 mg of base (26.3 mg of phosphate) daily for 2 weeks. If G6PD deficient, may have to give proguanil HCl continuously (100 mg daily) for 3 years.

HIV INFECTION

Attempts at specific treatment

Drug	Action
α interferon	Antiviral. Activates macrophages
γ interferon	Stimulates lymphokines
Interleukin-2	Proliferation B and T cells
Zidovudine	Inhibits reverse transcriptase

CYTOMEGALOVIRUS TREATMENT

Ganciclovir is related to acyclovir and is used to treat CMV infections in immunocompromised patients.
Foscarnet is indicated for CMV retinitis in patients with AIDS in whom ganciclovir is contraindicated.

Table 48 Antifungal agents — 1. Polyenes (bind to fungal cell membrane sterols to increase permeability, leakage of cell constituents and cell death)

Drug	General properties	Clinical use
Nystatin	Mainly for *Candida albicans*, but effective against other yeasts and fungi. Too toxic for systemic use so limited to superficial infections — topically not toxic or allergenic. Not absorbed from gut. Can be inhaled as aerosol for pulmonary infections and injected into cavities around a mycetoma without systemic absorption. Very safe — nausea if oral dose >5 million U/day Nystatin ointment, cream gel and dusting powder (100 000 U/g)	Used in intestinal and vaginal candidiasis. Effective in oropharyngeal candidosis but nasty taste.
Amphotericin B	More powerful action than nystatin against yeasts and fungi. Tolerated well topically and orally. Not absorbed from gut. Can be given systemically but toxic. High protein binding; poor penetration into body fluids. *Toxicity*: Renal damage common (reversible if drug stopped early and i.v. mannitol given). Headache, chills, hypotension. Drug fever (give 50 mg cortisol i.v.). Anaemia. Vomiting (give chlorpromazine 50 mg). Hypokalaemia.	Systemic mycoses — must be started early. Fungal meningitis. Mycotic joint infections. Oesophageal candidosis. Reduction of carriage of yeasts in gut

Table 49 Antifungal agents — 2 Non-polyenes

Drug	General properties	Clinical use
Flucytosine	Interferes with fungal RNA and DNA synthesis. Narrow spectrum synthetic antifungal — but effective against candida, cryptococcus. Ineffective against filamentous fungi (e.g. aspergillosis). Well absorbed from gut and widely distributed in body fluids including CSF. Low protein binding. Can be used with amphotericin B and imidazoles. Resistance can develop during treatment: little toxicity at levels below 100 µg/ml serum; above this can cause depression of marrow and liver function. Cumulation in renal failure	Can be used in systemic yeast infections (if strain is sensitive): particularly candida infections in immuno-suppressed patients and cryptococcal meningitis. Given with amphotericin B to prevent emergence of resistant organisms which occurs rapidly when flucytosine given alone

Table 49 (continued)

Drug	General properties	Clinical use
Imidazoles:	Inhibit ergosterol synthesis in cell membrane, block peroxidase	
Miconazole	Usually applied locally but can also be given i.v. (for systemic candida and coccidioides immitis). Parenterally has mild toxic effects similar to amphotericin. ? Potentiates warfarin	Oral candidosis skin infections by candida and dermatophytes. Fungal infections of oropharynx and GI
Fluconazole	Gastrointestinal upset, rash	Systemic candidosis
Itraconazole	Gastrointestinal upset, rash	and coccidioides, vaginal candidosis, tinea, Cryptococcal infections, Aspergillus infections.
Ketoconazole	Well absorbed from stomach if pH< 3. Does not enter CSF. Elevation liver enzymes, rashes, gynaecomastia	Systemic aspergillosis (given as oral capsules or i.v.). Tinea — all forms. Chronic mucocutaneous candidosis
Griseofulvin	Inhibits polymerisation of tubular protein into microtubules in fungi at mitosis. Well absorbed from gut (especially with fatty food). Low plasma levels but concentrated in keratin. Effective in dermatophyte infections. Not effective against yeasts or topically. *Toxicity*: headache, nausea and vomiting, potentiates action of alcohol. Contraindicated in porphyria and in serious lung disease. Decreases efficacy of coumarin anticoagulants	Indicated for dermatophyte infections which have not responded to topical treatment
Terbinafine	An allylamine which is given orally for dermatophytosis	Ringworm not suitable for local treatment. Not effective in pityriasis versicolor

Other imidazoles include Econozole and Clotrimazole, which are used locally for tinea and skin and genital candidosis

Table 50 Antiviral drugs

Drug	Mechanism of action	Clinical use	Adverse effects
Inosine Pranobex	Antimetabolite	Oral treatment for herpes zoster. Efficacy not proven.	Gout
Idoxuridine	Antimetabolite	Herpes zoster and herpes simplex. Genital herpes. Herpes simplex eye infections.	Avoid contact of conc. solutions with mucous membranes. Too toxic for systemic use
Acyclovir	Phosphorylated by specific enzyme in herpes infected cells then inhibits herpes DNA-polymerase 10–30 × more than host DNA- polymerase	Herpes simplex corneal ulcers Herpes simplex and zoster in immuno- compromised patients. Herpes encephalitis. Genital herpes	Raised urea and creatinine. Inflammation if extravasates. Reduce dose in renal failure
Amantadine	Interferes with uncoating of virus prior to cell penetration	Prophylaxis and reduction of severity of influenza A in vulnerable patients. Possible benefit in herpes zoster	CNS: Confusion, excitement, hallucinations (NB has an amphetamine-like action)
Zidovudine	Phosphorylated to triphosphate which inhibits viral reverse transcriptase	Prophylaxis of HIV infection when CD4 lymphocyte count falling	Anaemia, neutropenia, nausea, headache, rash, myalgia.

18. Cancer chemotherapy

DEFINITIONS

Doubling time — time for tumour to double cell number.
Cell cycle time — time for cell to go through cell cycle.
Growth fraction (G_F) — proportion of tumour in cell cycle. This fraction may be very large (75–80%) in small tumours which are thus sensitive to treatments which kill dividing cells.

Slow growth implies long period of tumour growth before clinical presentation — as tumour grows doubling time increases and G_F decreases.

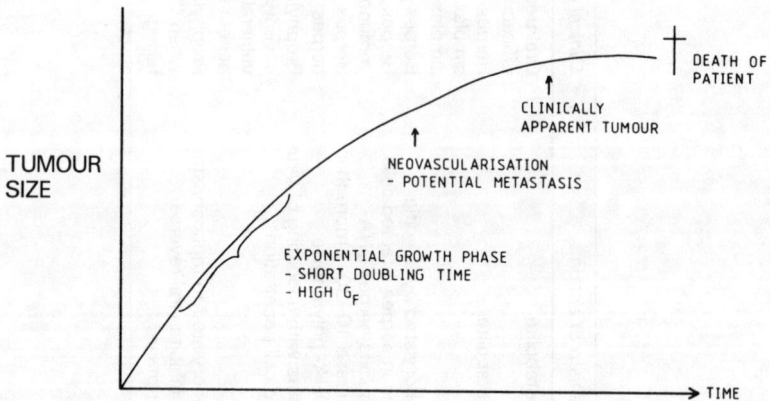

Fig. 18.1 Natural history of growth of a tumour.

No. of doublings	0	10	20	30	40
No. of cells	10^0	10^3	10^6	10^9	10^{12}
Tumour weight	0	1 μg	1 mg	1 g	1 kg

234

Note:
1. Clinical presentation of tumours is late — after about 30 doublings — death occurs after only another 10 doublings.
2. Metastasis occurs early — 1 mg tumour burden.

High G_F means greater tumour sensitivity to drugs so small tumours most likely to yield to chemotherapy (hence sometimes 'debulk' tumour with surgery/DXT before chemotherapy).

Curative chemotherapy must reduce tumour cells to nil or to such low numbers that body defences can kill rest. Aim is to allow more rapid recovery of normal cells whilst killing cancer cells by pulsed therapy.

Before treatment, tumours should be staged so that the best method of treatment and prognosis can be gauged from published reports. The objectives of treatment are thus defined. Drugs may have to be discontinued or substituted if the target responses are not attained. No mode of treatment is effective in all patients.

Drug combinations given as intermittent pulses:
1. Each drug of mixture has different toxicity so each used in optimal dose.
2. Each acts at different biochemical site.
3. Combination is additive to synergistic.
4. Some agents chosen to penetrate certain site, e.g. CNS.

If there is no evidence of benefit from combinations, then single drugs are used.

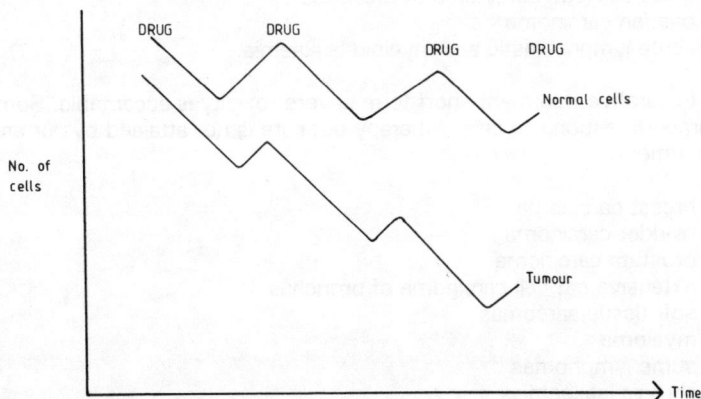

Fig. 18.2 This shows the effect of pulsed chemotherapy, which allows normal cells to recover in between treatments, but tumour cells are progressively reduced.

Clinical remission does not indicate cure: treatment for inapparent disease and micrometastases is needed — adjuvant or maintenance therapy. Cycle or phase-specific drugs useful here because micrometastases have high G_F — if non-cycle dependent drugs used dose must be low to avoid toxicity.

May be necessary to prevent recurrence from tumour nest in *sanctuary site* (immune from drug penetration), e.g. CNS, testis by specific drug therapy, e.g. inject methotrexate into CSF.

Adjuvant chemotherapy — to destroy disseminated microfoci of malignancy when no clinical evidence of residual disease is present after local treatment, but where it is known that relapses are common. This treatment is only used when evidence of possible benefit has been established by clinical trials. In stage II breast cancer, following operation 65% of women develop metastatic disease. Chemotherapy with cyclophosphamide, methotrexate and 5-fluorouracil (CMF) reduces this relapse rate by 20%.

Chemotherapy before local treatment (neo adjuvant chemotherapy) is used for some tumours, such as osteogenic sarcomas.

Treatment of established disease
Currently 80% of cancer chemotherapy is not curative but is to reduce symptoms and prolong disease-free and overall survival. Curative treatment is more likely in rapidly growing tumours in children and young adults. These include:

Hodgkin's disease and some non-Hodgkin's lymphomas
testicular seminoma and teratoma
choriocarcinoma
small cell (oat) carcinoma of bronchus
ovarian carcinoma
acute lymphoblastic and myeloid leukaemia.

In curative treatment short term severe toxicity is acceptable. Some tumours respond to chemotherapy but cure is not attained by current treatment:

breast carcinoma
bladder carcinoma
prostate carcinoma
extensive oat cell carcinoma of bronchus
soft tissue sarcomas
myeloma
some lymphomas
chronic leukaemias

Here very toxic chemotherapy is not acceptable. Chemotherapy is not routinely used for tumours which are generally unresponsive such as gastrointestinal and non-oat cell lung cancers.

Before chemotherapy, consider and assess: FBC; organ function (e.g. renal function before cisplatin); drug compatability factors.

Assessment of response
Chemotherapy is only carried out in a specialised hospital clinic. The response is monitored by observing symptoms, physical signs and repeated biochemical or radiological investigations. The duration of treatment is determined by established protocols and by the patient's response and usually involves 2 or more cycles of treatment after complete remission has been attained.

Toxic effects of cancer chemotherapy
1. Bone marrow
   — leucopenia; thrombocytopenia; rarely anaemia or total aplasia
   — immunosuppression and infections.
2. GI tract
   — nausea and vomiting
   — ulceration of mouth and intestine
   — diarrhoea.
3. Testis
   — azoospermia.
4. Ovary
   — infertility; premature menopause.
5. Hair follicles
   — alopecia.
6. Induction of second malignancies — e.g. acute myeloid leukaemia, non-Hodgkin's lymphoma.
7. Hyperuricaemia due to rapid tumour lysis.

Many drugs also locally irritant or have special toxicity.

Intrathecal injections. Only certain drugs can be given intrathecally to treat or prevent meningeal involvement. Vesicant drugs (such as mustards, vinca, daunorubicin) are lethal if injected intrathecally. Thus intravenous drugs must not be prepared, drawn up or administered at the same time as intrathecal drugs.

Cytotoxic drug handling. Only trained personnel should prepare drugs for administration. Protective clothing and eye protection should be worn and preparation take place only in designated areas. Pregnant women should not handle these drugs. Care should be taken in disposing of unused drugs and patients' excreta.

DRUGS USED IN CANCER CHEMOTHERAPY

Various groups:
1. Alkylating agents
2. Anti-metabolites

3. Plant alkaloids
4. Anti-tumour antibiotics
5. Random synthetics and enzymes
6. Hormones.

1. ALKYLATING AGENTS

Act via reactive alkyl ($R\text{-}CH_2\text{-}CH_2^+$) groups which react with nucleic acids (also proteins, enzymes) and inhibit function.

Cyclophosphamide

Mode of action
Not itself cytotoxic — activated in vitro by mainly hepatic microsomal enzymes to several reactive metabolites.

Adverse effects
Nausea and vomiting (50%) — frequently occurs following day, may last 72 h.
    Alopecia — particularly in the young (? because hair grows rapidly). Regrowth sometimes during treatment usual — takes 6–9 months.
    Cystitis — drink 2 l/water/day for at least 48 h after drug and empty bladder frequently. Bladder irrigation with cysteine may help. MESNA can prevent urotoxicity.
    Myelosuppression at 7–10 days — platelets relatively spared.

Ifosfamide
Isomer of cyclophosphamide activated to some of the same active metabolites but also some different ones. Has less myelosuppressant but greater renal toxic effects. Only used i.v. for lung, pancreatic, testicular cancer.

Other alkylating agents
Other commonly used alkylating agents are busulphan, melphalan, chlorambucil, mustine (nitrogen mustard), lomustine (CCNU), and carmustine.
    Thiotepa is mainly used as an intracavitary drug. Estramustine is a combination of oestrogen and mustine, and delivers mustine to oestrogen receptors e.g. in prostatic cancer. Treosulphan is used for ovarian cancer.
    The alkylating drugs generally severely inhibit gametogenesis and prolonged use (especially with X-irradiation) greatly increase the risk of developing leukaemia. Myelosuppression is the dose-limiting side effect.

2. ANTIMETABOLITES

Compounds which interfere with the utilisation of a natural metabolite (esp. nucleic acid or steroid).

Methotrexate

Mode of action
Inhibits dihydrofolate reductase.

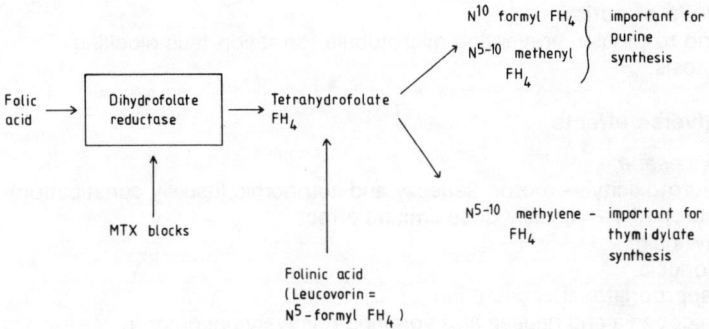

Fig. 18.3

Adverse effects (may be increased if renal function impaired and if NSAID concurrently given):
Myelosuppression
Gastro-intestinal mucositis; nausea and vomiting
Hepatitis and cirrhosis with chronic oral therapy (e.g. for psoriasis)
Nephrotoxicity
Neurotoxicity mainly after intrathecal injection.
(after treatment folinic acid administration — folinic acid rescue — prevents tissue toxicity).

Uses
Chorioncarcinoma
Acute lymphatic leukaemia
Osteogenic sarcoma.

Mercaptopurine and azathioprine are purine antimetabolites. Allopurinol greatly increases their actions.

Fluorouracil and cytarabine interfere with pyrimidine synthesis.

Mercaptopurine is used for maintenance therapy of acute leukaemias.

Thioguanine and cytarabine are used to induce remission and maintenance in acute myeloid leukaemia.

Azathioprine is mainly used as an immunosuppressant.

Bone marrow suppression is dose-limiting with the above antimetabolites.

3. PLANT ALKALOIDS

Vinca alkaloids
Derived from periwinkle plant (Vinca rosea): vincristine; vinblastine; vindesine.

Mode of action
Bind to tubulin, preventing microtubule formation thus blocking mitosis.

Adverse effects

Vincristine:
Neurotoxicity — motor, sensory and autonomic (usually constipation) neuropathy — usually dose-limiting effect
Jaw pain
Alopecia
Inappropriate ADH secretion
Leucopenia and nausea and vomiting relatively uncommon.

Vinblastine:
Myelosuppression nadir at 7–10 days (leucopenia >thrombocytopenia) — usually dose-limiting effect
Phlebitis
Alopecia
Neurotoxicity does occur but is uncommon.

Vindesine:
Side effects intermediate between vincristine and vinblastine.

Uses
Acute leukaemias
Hodgkin's and non-Hodgkin's lymphoma
Wilms tumour
Neuroblastoma.

Etoposide and teniposide
Alkaloid from mandrake plant.
   Spindle poison preventing cells entering mitosis. Binds to tubulin but probably acts by inhibiting topoisomerase.
   Can be given orally or i.v. $T_{1/2} = 11.5$ h.
   Dose limiting adverse effect is myelosuppression (nadir at 10–15 d) with nausea, vomiting and reversible alopecia also common.
   Active in small cell lung cancer; also lymphomas and testicular teratoma.

4. ANTITUMOUR ANTIBIOTICS

Act by intercalating in DNA helix or binding to DNA and interfering with transcription.

Doxorubicin (Adriamycin)
Anthracycline antibiotic produced by *Streptomyces peucetius*.
Intercalates DNA helix thus uncoiling and preventing DNA and RNA
synthesis.

Adverse effects
Irritant — avoid contact with skin or eyes and extravasation. Must be
given by fast-flowing i.v. infusion to avoid venous irritation and
cardiac arrhythmias.

Myelosuppression — 12–14 days after dose (later than many
cytotoxics).

Cardiotoxicity — dose-related cardiomyopathy with cardiomegaly
and cardiac failure. Total doses >550 mg/m^2 associated with
20–30% risk cardiotoxicity. If mediastinal radiotherapy or
cyclophosphamide used dose should not exceed 450 mg/m^2.

Nausea and vomiting common, may be moderate to severe.

Alopecia — common and often total if used with
cyclophosphamide. Head cooling may prevent but is cumbersome.

Radiation-recall phenomenon — erythema and skin oedema in skin
previously irradiated.

Red urine passed after drug (not haematuria!).

Uses
Hodgkin's and non-Hogkin's lymphomas, acute leukaemias and
several solid tumours including breast cancer.

Mitozantrone has similar structure and cardiotoxicity to doxorubicin.

Aclarubicin and **idarubicin** also resemble doxorubicin.

Other commonly used antitumour antibiotics are actinomycin D,
bleomycin, daunorubicin, epirubicin and mitomycin. Myelosuppression
is their dose-limiting toxicity — the nadir of granulocytes and platelets
is 10–15 d after treatment (apart from mitomycin which has a nadir at
28 d). Mucositis is also maximal at 10–15 d.

These antibiotics, potentiate the local effects of radiation, and
'radiation recall' may develop with drugs months after radiation.

Bleomycin is used to treat lymphomas. Dermatological toxicity is
common but dose-related pulmonary fibrosis is its main problem.

Actinomycin D is used for paediatric cancers. Its toxicity is similar to
that of doxorubicin but it is not cardiotoxic.

Mitomycin is used for gastrointestinal and breast cancers.

5. RANDOM SYNTHETICS AND ENZYMES

Procarbazine
Depolymerises DNA without affecting double helix structure.
Requires activation to azo-derivative.
  Rapid and almost complete GI absorption.

Adverse effects
Dose-related myelosuppression (nadir 7–10 days).
  Nausea and vomiting initially but less prominent after several doses.
  Procarbazine is weak, MAOI-food interactions rare but alcohol causes purplish facial flush. Care with tricyclic antidepressants, sympathomimetics and CNS depressants.

Uses
Hodgkin's disease, as in MOPP (mustine, vincristine, prednisolone and procarbazine).

Cisplatin
Platinum diaminodichloride — heavy metal coordination compound (expensive); only inorganic compound used in cancer chemotherapy.
Relatively selective DNA synthesis inhibitor.

Adverse effects
Vomiting and diarrhoea 2–4 h after starting drug and severe for several hours — may last for up to a week.
  Nephrotoxicity: dose-related, cumulative, irreversible tubular necrosis. Intravenous fluid loading is mandatory and renal function must be monitored.
  Ototoxicity: high tone deafness (up to 30% patients) ±tinnitus. May be irreversible.
  Myelosuppression: dose-related and cumulative especially with radiotherapy or other chemotherapy.
  Others: neuropathy, rashes, hypomagnesaemia.

Uses
Testicular and ovarian cancer.
Possibly bladder and head and neck cancers.

Carboplatin is as effective as cisplatin, but is less nephrotoxic and causes less nausea.

6. HORMONES

May produce remission in some cancers but do not eradicate disease.

1. Oestrogen used for 2 cancers which are partially hormone-dependent

a. Prostatic carcinoma
Oestrogens block androgen production with remission in 60% patients with advanced disease.

Main adverse effects are nausea, fluid retention (hypertension, oedema, heart failure), thromboembolism, feminisation and loss of libido.

Gonadotrophin releasing hormone (GnRH) analogues include buserilin, goserilin and leuprorelin. They are as effective as orchidectomy or stilboestrol.

b. Breast cancer

Oestrogens give remission in 30% women with advanced disease who are 5 years post-menopausal but may exacerbate disease in younger women. Tumours with oestrogen receptors 6 times more likely to respond (60%) than receptor negative tumours (10%). Hormone responsiveness inversely proportional to tumour aggressiveness; tumours metastates only to skin or bone have 30% response but lung or liver metastases show 10% response.

Diethylstilboestrol 1–15 mg/day in divided doses.

Adverse effects

Nausea

Fluid retention

Hypercalcaemia — serum Ca^{++} may rise rapidly especially with bony metastases.

2. Anti-oestrogens for breast cancer

a. Tamoxifen

Competes with oestradiol for cytoplasmic receptor. Few side effects and as effective as diethylstilboestrol. Dose 10 mg 12-hourly. Main toxicity: nausea; secondary to anti-oestrogen effect (hot flushes; occasional vaginal bleeding and pruritus). It is used in metastatic disease and as adjuvant treatment after surgery.

b. Aminoglutethimide

Produces medical adrenalectomy making surgery unnecessary and inhibits peripheral tissue aromatisation of androgens to oestrogens.

Reduction in cortisol produces rise in ACTH so 250 mg 6-hourly given with cortisone acetate 25 mg 12-hourly + fludrocortisone

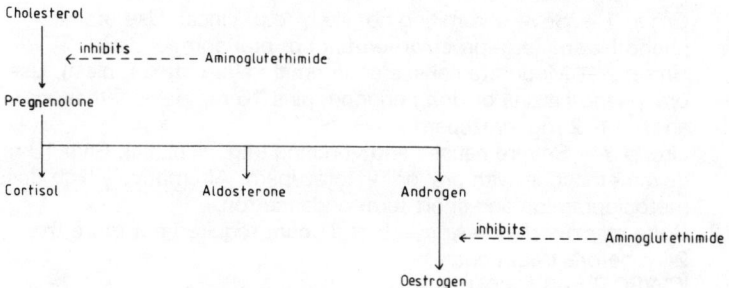

Fig. 18.4

0.1 mg alternate days (replaces aldosterone deficit). Side effects: lethargy, ataxia, dizziness (dose dependent and reduces with chronic therapy — self-induction of metabolising enzymes).
Rash sometimes with fever — usually self-limiting.

3. Prednisolone
Inhibits lymphoid proliferation. Dose 10–100 mg p.o. daily. Adverse effects numerous (see page 190). Used in acute and chronic lymphocytic leukaemia; multiple myeloma; Hodgkin's and non-Hodgkin's lymphomas; breast carcinoma.

Biological response modifiers
Interferons have activity against hairy cell leukaemia. Interleukin 2 has caused regression in some solid tumours, such as renal carcinoma.

Longer term hazards of cancer chemotherapy
1. Gonadal damage — alkylating agents, vinca alkaloids, cytosine arabinoside. Azoospermia usual during treatment. Recovery often occurs but may take several years (NB many patients have low sperm count before treatment). Many women develop amenorrhoea after cytotoxic drugs but periods restart when treatment stopped. Women in later 30s–40s may have premature menopause.
2. Second malignancy, e.g. after treatment of Hodgkins lymphoma with radio- and chemotherapy incidence of acute leukaemia increased 29-fold.
3. Teratogenesis: avoid pregnancy for at least 4 months after end of chemotherapy (in male and female).

Treatment of side effects and complications common to cytotoxic drugs
1. *Vomiting* — practical problem — treatment only about 70% effective. Injection usually given ½–1 hour before chemotherapy then continued or changed to oral therapy if no vomiting.
   Group 1 — Severe vomiting not likely (e.g. vinca). Use oral phenothiazine (e.g. prochlorperazine) or oral domperidone.
   Group 2 — Moderate nausea and vomiting (e.g. doxorubicin). Use oral phenothiazine or domperidone, plus 10 mg dexamethasone and/or 1–2 mg lorazepam.
   Group 3 — Severe nausea and vomiting (e.g. cisplatin). Give 10 mg dexamethasone with oral or i.v. lorazepam. Alternatively high dose metoclopramide and short term ondansetron.
2. *Bone marrow depression* — Blood count required not more than 24 h before treatment.
   If WBC $2.5–3.5 \times 10^9/l$ } halve dosage.
      Platelets $50–100 \times 10^9/l$ }

If WBC <2.5–10^9/l
   Platelets <50 × 10^9/l } without treatment
Patients with 0.8 × 10^9/l neutrophils and platelet counts
>4.0 × 10^9/l require only observation — below this admission and
antibiotic administration.
Platelet transfusions often needed if count <2.0 × 10^9/l
3. *Hyperuricaemia* — rare with solid tumours but common in
leukaemia and Hodgkin's disease. Given allopurinol before therapy
+ high fluid intake.

19. Drugs and the eye

GLAUCOMA

Increased intra-ocular pressure with impaired vision.
Two types of primary glaucoma — entirely different diseases:

1. OPEN ANGLE GLAUCOMA (CHRONIC SIMPLE GLAUCOMA)

Generally painless chronic condition with slow progressive visual loss.
Due to imbalance of *secretion* of aqueous (from ciliary epithelium) into
posterior chamber, and *outflow* from anterior chamber (usually
resistance to outflow lies in trabecular meshwork of angle or in cells
of canal of Schlemm). Drugs used chronically to normalise intra-ocular
pressure.

Treatment
Lowering of intra-ocular pressure in established disease: aim to lower
pressure below 21 mmHg throughout 24 h.

1. *Topical preparations*
    a. *β-blockers* applied locally are effective on a twice daily basis
       and rarely cause ocular unwanted effects. Timolol is absorbed
       sufficiently to aggravate asthma, heart failure and bradycardia.
       Carteolol and betaxolol have less systemic toxicity, but still
       cause bronchial obstruction in asthmatics. Metipranolol is
       similar to timolol, but cheaper.
    b. *Parasympatheticomimetics*: constrict pupil and reduce
       resistance to outflow of aqueous by increasing tension in
       scleral spur, thereby opening up the trabeculae around
       Schlemm's canal. The drugs include pilocarpine, neostigmine
       and ecothiopate.
    c. Drugs acting on the sympathetic system:
       Adrenaline 1 and 2% eye drops (Eppy) — useful addition to
       pilocarpine especially in early cataract by allowing a larger pupil.
       Adrenaline reduces resistance to outflow (α-effect) and reduces
       secretion of aqueous (β-effect). The benefit of adrenaline is
       further increased by the addition of *guanethidine* drops (3 or
       5%).

Problems with adrenaline:
— red eye as effect wears off
— conjunctival pigmentation
— irritation.
Dipivefrine is a prodrug of adrenaline which rapidly passes through the cornea.

2. Oral drugs

Acetazolamide (Diamox): inhibits carbonic anhydrase responsible for aqueous secretion.

Given as 125 mg 8-hourly or 500 mg (Diamox Sustets) 12-hourly in open angle glaucoma with local treatment.

Adverse effects:
— diuresis — short-lived (few days) as acid-base status changes but
  effect on aqueous formation continues
— paraesthesiae
— indigestion and nausea
— depression.

Dichlorphenamide — carbonic anhydrase inhibitor used if acetazolamide side effects troublesome.

Methyldopa can dangerously lower perfusion pressure in optic nerve head.
Systemic β-blockers can help to relieve glaucoma.

2. ANGLE-CLOSURE GLAUCOMA

Due to occlusion of the filtration angle by the iris root coming into contact with the peripheral cornea.
a. Acute angle-closure glaucoma is an ophthalmic emergency which presents as a red and painful eye associated with photophobia and visual loss.

Drugs used to control pressure prior to surgery.

Treatment
1. *Dehydrating agents*: intravenous infusions of hypertonic solutions
   of urea, mannitol, glycerol. Glycerol also given orally. Produce
   diuresis and dehydration of tissues.
2. *Oral acetazolamide* in high doses, e.g. 250 mg 6-hourly.
3. *Topical miotics*: pilocarpine used to prevent mydriasis *after*
   lowering of intraocular pressure has been attained in patients with
   a fixed pupil. Pilocarpine is given early when the pupil is not fixed.
4. *Analgesics* e.g. pethidine, morphine, may be required to control
   pain.

5. *Iridectomy* is performed after the coincidental inflammation has settled.

b. Primary chronic (creeping) angle-closure glaucoma.
Avoid precipitating factors:
   Pupil dilating drugs — local and systemic atropine-like agents contraindicated in closed angle glaucoma but have no harmful effect in chronic simple glaucoma.
   Steroid applied to the eye can raise ocular pressure in some individuals and worsen glaucoma.
   Acute angle-closure glaucoma can arise in chronic angle-closure glaucoma and require urgent treatment.

UVEITIS

The uveal tract is derived from the mesoderm surrounding the optic cup. It comprises the iris, ciliary body and choroid. Uveitis may be secondary to external trauma or arise due to systemic diseases.
   Blindness results from obliteration of pupil aperture, secondary glaucoma, cataract and macular involvement.
1. Specific treatment of cause when possible.
2. Local and systemic steroids (except in infective uveitis due to Herpes simplex or zoster).
      Local steroid eye preparations include:
      betamethasone disodium phosphate 0.1% drops and ointment — application may be as frequent as hourly
      clobetasone butyrate 0.1% drops ⎫ have least effect on
      fluoromethalone 0.1% suspension ⎭ intraocular pressure
      prednisolone sodium phosphate 0.5% drops
      In severe inflammation a sub-conjunctival injection of methylprednisolone acetate (Depo-Medrone) gives a high anterior chamber steroid concentration over several days. Oral prednisolone (60–100 mg) is used systemically.
NB Steroids should *never* be used indiscriminately in the eye as use in infection (bacterial or viral) encourages infective spread within the eye.
3. Occasionally increased intra-ocular tension + thinning of the cornea due to steroids ruptures the globe.
4. Azathioprine or oxyphenbutazone (10% ointment) can be applied locally to reduce steroid dose.
5. The pupil is maintained dilated.

EYE INFECTIONS

Treatment often started before pathogen identified using clinical picture as a guide.
   May need to change antibacterial within first 48 h.

Antibacterials given in 4 ways:
1. Drops
   — for superficial infections, e.g. conjunctivitis
   — need to give 2-hourly because tears dilute drug.
2. Ointments
   — release drug more slowly especially if eye covered with pad.
3. Subconjunctival injection (0.5–1 ml) gives therapeutic levels for 8–12 hours.
4. Systemic administration
   — used for deep or posterior segment infections
   — drug penetration variable, e.g. ampicillin, chloramphenicol, have good penetration especially in inflammation.

a. *Broad spectrum agents:*
Chloramphenicol (0.5% eye drops or 1% ointment).
Neomycin sulphate (eye drops BNF or 0.25% ointment).
Framycetin sulphate (0.5% ointment) — effective against pseudomonas.

b. *Other agents:*
Sulphacetamide (eye drops 30%) has been used for trachoma but tetracycline hydrochloride 1% eye ointment is now the treatment of choice.

Penicillin is used in gonococcal ophthalmia neonatorum.

(Chloramphenicol is used for most other forms of conjunctivitis in the newborn and tetracycline or sulphacetamide for TRIC agent conjunctivitis).

Bacterial infections often produce damage by inflammatory response rather than bacterial toxicity. Steroids often used with antibiotics (but rarely in conjunctivitis unless there is specific indication because of danger of exacerbating infection). Various steroid/anti-infective drugs available, e.g. betamethasone 0.1% + neomycin sulphate 0.5% (Betnesol-N) are available.

Herpes simplex infections treated with:
Idoxuridine (0.1%) drops applied hourly in day and 2-hourly at night or ointment (0.5%) — 4 times daily.

Experts use steroids with antiviral agents to limit damage.
NB Herpid (5% idoxuridine in dimethyl sulphoxide) is for use on skin NOT eyes which it may damage.
Vidarabine 3% (Vira-A) ointment applied 5 times daily
or Acyclovir 3% ointment (Zovirax) applied 4-hourly also useful in herpes.

Anti-inflammatory preparations
Topical anti-histamines as drops are used in allergic conjunctivitis, e.g. antazoline sulphate 0.5% + xylometazoline hydrochloride 0.05% (Otrivine-Antistin). Sodium cromoglycate 2% drops (Opticrom) used as prophylactic 4 times daily.

DRUGS WHICH HARM THE EYE

1. Tricyclic antidepressants and anticholinergic anti-Parkinsonian drugs:
   Failure of accommodation
   Aggravation of angle-closure glaucoma.
2. Phenothiazine neuroleptics:
   Pigmentary retinopathy (especially thioridazine)
   Anterior polar cataract (especially chlorpromazine)
   Anticholinergic effects.
3. Glucocorticoids:
   Systemic steroids: Posterior subcapsular cataracts (rare if dose <10 mg prednisolone/day)
   Papilloedema (rare) due to raised intracranial pressure when steroid dose reduced — treat by raising steroid dose again
   Raised intra-ocular pressure (see above)
   Infections encouraged
   Local steroids: Can also raise intra-ocular pressure, cause cataract and can aggravate Herpes simplex corneal ulcers.
4. Chloroquine:
   Subepithelial linear corneal deposits (reversible)
   Retinal pigmentation, arteriolar damage and macular damage cause field defects and loss of central vision (irreversible).
5. Amiodarone:
   Corneal deposits — produce no visual impairment.
6. Ethambutol (more than 15 mg/kg/day):
   Optic neuritis (produces blindness) — more likely in alcoholics or diabetics.
7. Fetal damage to eye from taking the following during pregnancy:
   Thalidomide
   Phenytoin
   Busulphan.

20. Drug overdose

Approximately 10% of acute adult medical admissions are because of overdoses. Some evidence for increase over the past 20 years.
Causes in order of frequency:
1. parasuicide (manipulative self-poisoning)
2. suicidal intent (often associated with depression and schizophrenia)
3. accidental (commonest in children)
4. homicidal (very rare).

Long-term management requires the distinction between these groups to be made.
NB also rare group of children who have been deliberately overdosed by parents as manifestation of parent's mental illness.

Overdosage is commonly with more than one drug (alcohol is the commonest component) and thus the clinical features are variable.

Overdose mortality overall in hospital <1%.

Approximately 10% cases require treatment other than careful nursing.

MANAGEMENT

1. Diagnosis
2. Supportive therapy
3. Specific measures
4. Psychiatric.

1. DIAGNOSIS

   a. History from patient or companion:
      drug taken, alcohol taken in addition, treatment for other diseases, obvious signs in present illness, e.g. fits.
   b. Past history of psychiatric illness:
      suicide attempts
      drug abuse and alcoholism.
   c. Physical signs, for example:

Fits
   tricyclic antidepressants
   amphetamine, cocaine and other stimulants
   antihistamines
   narcotic analgesics
   neuroleptics
   solvents.
Pulmonary oedema
   narcotic analgesics
   glutethimide.
Skin bullae
   any cause of coma.
Papilloedema
   glutethimide.
Involuntary movements or restlessness
   salicylates
   antihistamines
   anticholinergics
   neuroleptics
   lithium
   tricyclic antidepressants.
Coma
   hypnosedatives
   alcohol
   narcotic analgesics
   tricyclic antidepressants.
Also look for jaundice, injection marks, scars, necrosis and gangrene.
   d. Special diagnostic procedures: drug screen in blood, urine and
      gastric contents. Look for mixtures (including alcohol). Retain
      sample for forensic purposes.
   e. Grade level of consciousness:
      I.   drowsy, responds to verbal commands
      II. unconscious but responds to minimally painful stimuli
      III. unconscious, responds only to very painful stimuli
      IV. unconscious, does not respond to stimuli.
   f. Monitor:
      respiratory functions: respiratory minute volume (if <4 l,
      then do arterial Po_2, Pco_2, pH and standard bicarbonate)
      circulatory: pulse rate and blood pressure
      temperature: rectal temperature measurment
      blood: urea, electrolytes, haematocrit
      renal function: urine output (bladder catheterisation required in
      severely poisoned patients).

2. SUPPORTIVE THERAPY

   a. Maintain airway and ventilation: most important initial
      procedure as respiratory failure is commonest immediate cause

of death. Respiratory stimulants are dangerous and should not be used.

b. Shock: treat with intravenous fluids (plasma, dextran) with monitoring of central venous pressure and clinical observation.

c. Hypothermia: contributes to shock, acidaemia and hypoxia and measurement of core temperature imperative.
Avoid active reheating.
Wrap patient in foil or 'space' blanket to conserve heat and nurse in warm atmosphere. Use warmed humidified air if on ventilator.

d. Treat cardiac arrhythmias.

e. Prolonged or repeated fits are controlled with intravenous diazepam.

f. Monitor and control fluid and electrolyte balance.

g. Nursing care of unconscious patient: regular turning, eye and mouth care, attention to pressure areas etc. very important.

3. SPECIFIC MEASURES

A. Prevention of further absorption

a. In a conscious child or adult, induce vomiting by irritation of pharynx with spatula. Alternatively give 15 ml syrup of ipecac which causes vomiting in 15–20 mins. Avoid apomorphine (causes protracted vomiting) and saline (causes electrolyte imbalance).

b. Gastric aspiration and lavage should be undertaken if known that drug ingested within previous 4 hours (exception salicylate, tricyclics and anticholinergics when it may be worthwhile at later times). Wide bore stomach tube is passed and 500 mg warm water repeatedly ($\times$ 5–8) introduced and emptied from stomach. All lavage fluid should be removed at end of washout except in iron poisoning when 10 g desferrioxamine is left in stomach.

Danger of aspiration pneumonia so protective gag reflex must be present before starting washout. If reduced or absent, washout is performed with a cuffed endotracheal tube in place.

Lavage can be traumatic and must be done cautiously if corrosive poisons taken. It is contraindicated in overdose with petroleum and related solvents.

It is impracticable in children.

c. Activated charcoal prevents the absorption of some drugs (e.g. tricyclic antidepressants) and may also enhance the elimination of drugs after they have been absorbed.

B. Enhancement of drug elimination

Applicable in few cases.

Reduces duration of coma and therefore of secondary complications like pneumonia, hypotension, thromboembolism.
Little trial evidence that overall outcome altered.

a. Forced diuresis
1. Alkaline diuresis:
— salicylates
— phenobarbitone, barbitone (only barbiturates that have sufficiently
 high renal excretion to make its enhacement worthwhile: others
 undergo hepatic metabolism).
Principle: To increase proportion of ionised drug in renal tubules thus
reducing tubular reabsorption since only lipophilic unionised molecules
cross cell membranes readily. Ionisation of acids is increased in
alkaline urine and vice versa.
Method:
a. Ascertain that:
   (i) BP adequate (i.e. patient not shocked)
   (ii) pulmonary oedema absent
   (iii) CVP line and peripheral venous line in place
   (iv) current electrolyte status is known
   (v) as far as possible that renal function normal.
b. Follow scheme on page 255 (Fig. 20.1).

NB This is a dangerous procedure — monitor JVP, lung bases, CVP
(chest X-ray) and electrolytes frequently. Discontinue as soon as drug
level has fallen adequately and patient's clinical condition improved.
2. Acid diuresis.
Rarely used for amphetamine and other bases. Urinary acidification
difficult to achieve because respiratory stimulation produces
consequent respiratory alkalosis.

b. Haemoperfusion
Passage of blood over column of activated charcoal or ion-exchange
resin via extracorporeal circuit.
   Used for barbiturates, glutethimide, chloral hydrate, meprobamate,
methaqualone, paracetamol, theophylline.
   Available only in specialist centres and danger of haemorrhage,
infection, platelet and leucocyte consumption on column, air
embolism.

c. Haemodialysis
Used for severe lithium intoxication, salicylate, methanol and ethylene
glycol poisioning.
NB Measurement of plasma drug concentration is only rarely
important in management but it is in these cases in which active
elimination measures are used where it is most useful.

Special features of particular drug overdoses
Only rarely is there a specific antidote for a given drug. Most patients
recover with simple nursing measures.
Benodiazepines, one of the commonest overdoses, exemplify this
approach. Flumazenil, a benzodiazepine antagonist is used to assist
diagnosis.

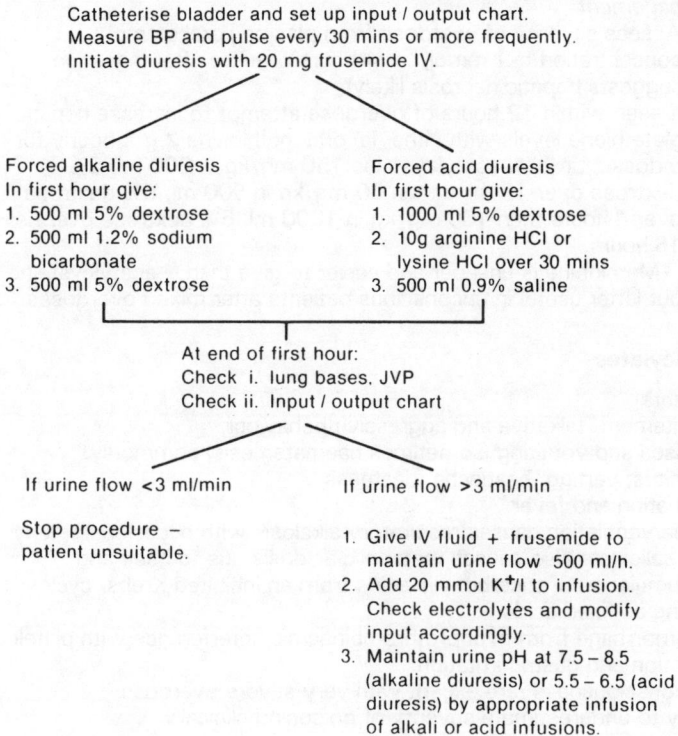

Catheterise bladder and set up input / output chart.
Measure BP and pulse every 30 mins or more frequently.
Initiate diuresis with 20 mg frusemide IV.

Forced alkaline diuresis
In first hour give:
1. 500 ml 5% dextrose
2. 500 ml 1.2% sodium
   bicarbonate
3. 500 ml 5% dextrose

Forced acid diuresis
In first hour give:
1. 1000 ml 5% dextrose
2. 10g arginine HCl or
   lysine HCl over 30 mins
3. 500 ml 0.9% saline

At end of first hour:
Check i. lung bases, JVP
Check ii. Input / output chart

If urine flow <3 ml/min

Stop procedure –
patient unsuitable.

If urine flow >3 ml/min

1. Give IV fluid + frusemide to
   maintain urine flow 500 ml/h.
2. Add 20 mmol K^+/l to infusion.
   Check electrolytes and modify
   input accordingly.
3. Maintain urine pH at 7.5 – 8.5
   (alkaline diuresis) or 5.5 – 6.5 (acid
   diuresis) by appropriate infusion
   of alkali or acid infusions.

Fig. 20.1

Paracetamol

Effects
Patient is conscious, but may be nauseated and vomit. Main hazard is
delayed hepatocellular necrosis after 2–3 days. As little as 10–15 g
may produce dangerous toxicity.

Mechanism of toxicity
In overdose, the usual metabolic pathway ($\rightarrow$ sulphate + glucuronide)
is overloaded and more drug is metabolised via mixed function
oxidase. Usually products of this minor pathway are detoxified by
glutathione, but in overdose this protective mechanism is
overwhelmed and reactive intermediates covalently combine with
hepatic intracellular enzymes and other proteins. Toxicity more likely if
patient's liver enzymes induced by other drugs.

Management
1. Assess severity of overdose from plasma paracetamol concentration (>1 mmol/l at 4 hours or more after ingestion suggests hepatic necrosis likely).
2. If seen within 12 hours of overdose attempt to increase hepatic glutathione levels with either (a) oral methionine 2 g 2-hourly for 5 doses, or (b) N-acetylcysteine 150 mg/kg in 200 ml, 5% dextrose over 15 mins then 50 mg/kg in 500 ml, 5% dextrose over 4 hours then 100 mg/kg in 1000 ml, 5% dextrose over next 16 hours.
   Methionine is cheaper and easier to give than N-acetylcysteine but latter useful in unconscious patients after mixed overdoses.

Salicylates

Effects
Excitement, talkative and aggressive behaviour.
Nausea and vomiting (sometimes haematemesis) commonly.
Tinnitus, vertigo, headache, deafness.
Sweating and fever.
Hyperventilation causes respiratory alkalosis with occasional tetany but salicylate also causes metabolic acidosis due to itself and accumulation of tricarboxylic acids from an inhibited Krebs' cycle acting as fixed acids.
Haemorrhage from hypoprothrombinaemia, interference with platelet function and gastric irritation.
Unconsciousness rare except with very severe overdose.
Easy to underestimate severity of poisoning clinically.

Management
1. Never too late to start gastric lavage.
2. Take blood for salicylate level. If >3.5 mmol/l consider forced alkaline diuresis (>2.2 mmol/l in children).
3. If abdominal pain give magnesium antacids.
4. In severe poisoning given 10 mg vitamin K i.m.

Opioids

Effects
Stupor and coma
Respiratory depression with cyanosis
Pinpoint pupils
Possibly pulmonary oedema and/or cardiac arrhythmias.

Management
1. Ventilate with oxygen, preferably via endotracheal tube to prevent aspiration.

2. Give naloxone 0.4 mg i.v., wait 3 mins, if no effect give 1.2 mg i.v., wait 3 mins, if no effect give 3.6 mg i.v. Repeat doses as required. Remember (a) naloxone $T_{1/2}$ effect shorter than opioids; (b) naloxone precipitates acute withdrawal reactions in opiate addicts.
3. Give i.v. glucose and thiamine in addicts.

Mixed opioid preparations
1. Co-proxamol (dextropropoxyphene + paracetamol) requires treatment with naloxone + methionine or N-acetylcysteine. Common overdose. Potentially very toxic (especially with alcohol).
2. Lomotil (diphenoxylate + atropine) Usually taken by children in overdose. Slowed gastric emptying delays narcotic effects for several hours so gastric lavage can often be useful several hours after ingestion. Treat with naloxone and symptomatic measures for anticholinergic effects.

Digitalis

Management
1. Maintain normal plasma K^+ by infusion (NB vomiting produces hypokalaemia).
2. Treat:
   bradycardia with atropine
   ventricular tachycardia with phenytoin.
3. Consider insertion of prophylactic pacemaker.
4. EDTA to lower plasma Ca^{++} rarely used.
5. Administration of digoxin antibodies has been found effective.

Barbiturates

Effects
Coma, sometimes with fluctuation of consciousness.
Dilated, unresponsive pupils, sometimes with flat EEG may be confused with brain death.
Respiratory depression and sudden apnoea.
Hypotension with shock and renal failure.
10% develop bullous eruption: no diagnostic value as occurs in other overdoses.

Management
1. Supportive
2. Phenobarbitone and barbitone only can be removed by forced alkaline diuresis.
3. Haemoperfusion effective in severe overdose.

β-adrenergic blockers

Effects

Bradycardia, hypotension, low cardiac output, conduction defects
in heart
Bronchospasm in asthmatics
Convulsions
Coma.

Management
1. Gastric lavage (even several hours after overdose).
2. Insert i.v. line, estimate blood gases and pH.
3. 500 mg cortisol i.v. initially.
4. If hypotensive give isoprenaline 10–20 µg/min i.v. If bradycardia
   give atropine 2 mg i.v. as a single dose, but a pacemaker may
   have to be inserted.
   If low cardiac output does not respond to isoprenaline, give
   glucagon (in dextrose) 5–15 mg/h i.v.
   If persistent hypotension give dopamine, dobutamine or
   noradrenaline.
   Persistent refractory low cardiac output may require an aortic
   balloon pump.
5. For bronchospasm i.v. or aerosol salbutamol.
6. Correct acidosis.
7. Correct fluid retention with frusemide.

Tricyclic antidepressants

Effects

Hyperreflexia; tremor; excitement; fits.
Supraventricular and ventricular tachycardias; intracardiac blocks;
   cardiac arrest can occur 4–6 days after overdose.
Anticholinergic effects: dilated pupils, paralytic ileus, retention of
   urine.
Coma, hypotension or hypertension, respiratory depression.

Management
1. Insert intravenous line.
2. Gastric lavage (even 1 day after overdose).
3. Put activated charcoal in stomach after lavage (25 g/g of drug
   ingested).
4. Repeated blood gas estimations (treat acidosis with i.v.
   bicarbonate but ventilate when required).
5. i.v. diazepam if repeated fits.
6. i.v. infusion of a plasma expander if hypotension due to peripheral
   circulatory failure.

7. Continuous cardiac monitoring (correction of hypoxia and acidosis may correct arrhythmias but treat persistent supraventricular tachycardia with propranolol); ventricular tachycardias with lignocaine or disopyramide; bradycardia with conduction defects requires insertion of a pacemaker.

Iron
Commonly in children who take their pregnant mother's iron tablets which resemble sweets.

Effects
Gastritis, vomiting, diarrhoea, haematemesis. This settles in 12–24 hours and patient becomes well but will develop hepatocellular necrosis, renal failure, cardiac damage, haemorrhagic enterocolitis, convulsions and coma after a further 12–24 hours.

Management
1. Gastric lavage using chelating agent desferrioxamine (see above).
2. Desferrioxamine 2 g i.m. then i.v. at not greater rate than 15 mg/kg/h (max 80 mg/kg/day).
3. Continue treatment until serum iron concentration <200 mmol/l or transferrin no longer 100% saturated.

4. PSYCHIATRIC ASSESSMENT

Patients should usually be seen by a psychiatrist prior to discharge from the medical unit. Approximately equal number of patients fall into the categories:
1. depressive illness
2. personality disorder (often 'repeat overdoses')
3. drug addicts and alcoholics
4. no psychiatric disorder (intolerable socio-economic pressures; unhappy love affair; adolescent tantrums, etc).
Not all of these will benefit from further psychiatric follow-up or social help.

Some specific antidotes for overdose

Drug	Antidote
Lithium	NaCl infusion
Monoamine oxidase inhibitors	Hypertensive reactions: α-blocker (e.g. chlorpromazine) Tachycardia: β-blocker
Coumarin anticoagulants	Water soluble analogues of vitamin K (e.g. menaphthone)

Cyanide	Dicobalt edetate 20 ml of 1.5% solution given over 1 minute *stat*. and 50 ml of 50% glucose i.v., *or* sodium nitrite 10 ml of 3% solution given i.v. over 3 minutes, then sodium thiosulphate 25 ml of 50% solution i.v.
Methanol	i.v. ethanol (e.g. 5% solution) slows down conversion to formaldehyde.
Organophosphorus anticholinesterases	Pralidoxime (30 mg/kg) in 5 ml water, slow i.v. injection, repeat after 1 min, *plus* atropine 2 mg i.v. followed by 1 mg i.v. every 10 mins until bradycardia and meiosis reversed.
Mercury and arsenic	D penicillamine up to 1.5 g/day oral *or* injection of BAL 2.5 mg every 4–6 hours for first day; 2 injections/day for next 3 days; then 1 injection daily until recovery.
Lead and copper	Calcium disodium edetate 15–25 mg/kg slow i.v. injection twice daily (as a 0.5–3% solution in 5% glucose) *or* BAL *or* penicillamine.

21. Drug dependence

Definition
State of chronic intoxication produced by repeated drug administration which is detrimental to individual and society. There is compulsion to continue taking the drug and individual may exhibit one or more of:
1. Tolerance — increasing amounts of drug required to produce same effect.
2. Physical dependence — body adapts to drug and abnormal reactions (withdrawal reactions) occur if drug administration stopped abruptly.
3. Psychic dependence — drug produces satisfaction and pleasure such as to require further administration to maintain the sense of pleasure or to avoid discomfort.

Characteristic features of drug dependence vary with drug. Caffeine (in tea, coffee, chocolate, cocoa, coca-cola) produces dependence with a physical withdrawal syndrome (headache, yawning, tiredness) but this is generally regarded as harmless.

WHO classification

Type	Compounds
Alcohol-barbiturate	Ethanol, barbiturates and other hypnotics and sedatives, e.g. benzodiazepines
Amphetamine	Amphetamine, dexamphetamine, methylamphetamine, methylphenidate and phenmetrazine
Cocaine	Cocaine and coca leaves, cocaine free base
Cannabis	Preparations of *Cannabis sativa*, e.g. marihuana and hashish
Opiates	Opium, morphine, heroin, methadone, pethidine, etc.
Hallucinogens	Lysergic acid diethylamide (LSD), mescaline and psilocybin
Volatile compounds	Acetone, carbon tetrachloride and other solvents, e.g. 'glue-sniffing'
Nicotine	Tobacco, snuffs

Alcohol
1 unit = a single of spirits = 1 glass of wine = ½ pint of beer.
1 unit of alcohol raises blood alcohol by 10 mg/100 ml.
Urinary concentration is 1.3 × blood concentration.

Acute intoxication
NB Rate limiting enzyme is alcohol dehydrogenase which can
metabolise about 10 g pure ethanol/hour (spirits about 50% ethanol).
Thus pharmacokinetics show saturation and rapid accumulation once
metabolic capacity exceeded.

1. Main CNS effects:
reduced judgment and discrimination
reduced learning and attention span
impaired body-mind-eye coordination
social disinhibition.

Blood level (mg/100 ml)	Usual result (but much individual variation: habitual drinkers exhibit reduced effects)
20	Feeling of warmth and relaxation
30	Mild relief from anxiety; facilitation of conversation
50	Incoordination; slowed reactions; speech mistakes
100	Ataxia; slurred speech
100–200	Vertigo; difficulty walking; vomiting
300	Stupor
400	Deep anaesthesia; respiratory depression

2. Other actions:
cutaneous and conjunctival vasodilatation
sweating
tachycardia
suppression of ADH production
increased gastric acid secretion; gastritis
metabolic and respiratory acidosis
hyperuricaemia
hypoglycaemia.

Chronic effects of alcohol
1. Nervous system:
  a. Dependence:
withdrawal states:
    tremor
    fits
    delirium tremens
    anxiety, insomnia, panic attacks.

    b. Chronic neuronal degeneration:
       cerebral atrophy — dementia
       cerebellar syndromes
       psychiatric syndromes, e.g. depression, paranoia
    c. Consequences of vitamin deficiency:
       Wernicke's encephalopathy (features of acute and/or
       chronic organic psychosis +
       ophthalmoplegia + nystagmus)
       Korsakoff's psychosis (amnesic syndrome)
       Pellagra dementia — nicotinic acid lack.
2. *Alimentary*:
   chronic gastritis; peptic ulcer
   haematemesis (ulcer, varices, gastritis, Mallory-Weiss
   syndrome)
   acute, sub-acute and chronic pancreatitis
   hepatitis; cirrhosis.
3. Myopathy.
4. Bone marrow suppression.
5. In some patients: hypertriglyceridaemia, hyperglycaemia, harm to
   fetus.
6. Gout and accelerated atherogenesis.

Fetal alcohol syndrome
CNS:
   mild to moderate mental retardation
   poor coordination, hypotonia
   irritability and hyperactivity.
Facial features:
   microcephaly
   short, upturned nose
   hypoplastic maxilla
   micrognathia
   thinned upper vermilion of lips
   retarded pre-natal and post-natal.
Growth:
   small baby.

Drug interactions
May have medico-legal implications:
1. Potentiation of central depressants:
   anticholinergics, e.g. atropine, benztropine
   antihistamines (H_1-receptor blockers)
   barbiturates and glutethimide
   benzodiazepines
   chloral
   codeine
   dextropropoxyphene
   mianserin

phenothiazines
propranolol (? other β-blockers)
tricyclic antidepressants
2. Disulfiram reaction (flushing, palpitations, tachycardia,
   hypotension, giddiness, nausea and vomiting)
   Disulfiram (use as Antabuse in aversion therapy)
   Metronidazole
   Sulphonylureas especially chlopropamide
   Procarbazine
   Moxalactam
   Cefamandole
   Griseofulvin (?)
   Trichlorethylene (industrial exposure).
3. Potentiates hypoglycaemia due to other agents.
4. Enzyme induction reduces action of some drugs, e.g.
   tolbutamide, warfarin, phenytoin, but liver metabolism reduced
   following a binge so action of drugs can be potentiated, e.g.
   phenylbutazone.
5. Enhanced gastic irritation by non-steroidal anti-inflammatory
   agents.
6. Brain sensitivity to benzodiazepines reduced in chronic alcoholics
   (cross tolerance).

Treatment of alcohol abstinence syndromes
Develops within hours of last drink, peaks 24–48 hours, gone at 3–4
days. Less than 10% progress to delirium tremens.
Characterised by tremor, tachycardia, gut upsets. In all but mild cases
treat in hospital. Use benzodiazepines with long $T\frac{1}{2}$ in large doses
(cross-tolerance with alcohol).

> Diazepam — 40 mg daily for 4 days
> 30 mg daily for 3 days
> 20 mg daily for 2 days
> 10 mg daily for 1 day

Chlormethiazole is also an excellent sedative, anxiolytic and
anticonvulsant but has an addiction risk. Lorazepam is useful if there is
serious hepatic dysfunction.
Chlorpromazine reduces panic but can precipitate fits and is thus
not recommended.
Also give Parenterovite ± folic acid.

Delirium tremens (DTs)
A serious physical illness accompanied by physical illusions and
hallucinations which are typically unpleasant and often visual (e.g.
small animals or insects crawling over body). There is profound
confusion and disorientation and terrifying nightmares ('the horrors').
Diazepam used as above or given intravenously (10 mg stat then
5 mg every 5 minutes until calm) supplemented with haloperidol

2–4 mg i.m. every 4–6 hours. Haloperidol can be discontinued without tapering dose.

Fluid and electrolyte balance may required adjustment.

Give vitamins including high-dose vitamin B complex.

Treat any concurrent illness, especially infections, which can precipitate DTs.

Physical restraint occasionally required to protect patient and staff.

Rum fits
Grand mal seizures 7–48 hours after drinking stopped (~5% develop status).

i.v. diazepam treatment of choice.

Check Mg^{++} level — give 1 g MgSO$_4$ i.m. four times daily for 2 days prophylactically.

Overall treatment
Also requires:
1. Counselling and attention to behavioural and social factors.
2. Treatment of any underlying psychiatric disorder, e.g. depression
3. Group therapy (as with Alcoholics Anonymous).
4. Follow-up.

A few patients are helped by aversion therapy using disulfiram or other alcohol sensitising drugs.

Barbiturates and other hypnosedatives
Taken orally, i.v. or subcutaneously.

Chronic abuse
Drowsiness
Ataxia, nystagmus
Reduced quality and quantity of work
Increased appetite.

Withdrawal
Anxiety
Insomnia
Panic attacks
Fits (sometimes status epilepticus).

Benzodiazepines
Can cause the same picture as barbiturate 3–13 days after stopping drug.

Patients at risk usually on large doses (5–10 times therapeutic) for several months but few cases described after therapeutic dose.

Treatment
Stop benzodiazepine gradually.
Replace with 40 mg propranolol 8-hourly for 2 weeks.

Amphetamine and cocaine
Taken orally i.v. or sniffed (cocaine).
These have similar effects — both have central catecholamine effects.
Psychic dependence only.

Acute administration
Excitement, euphoria, little need for sleep
Anorexia
Psychotic schizophrenia-like reactions, sometimes violent tremor,
Tachycardia, dangerous arrhythmias
Hypertension
Fits.

Withdrawal
Depression
Hyperphagia
Hypersomnia.
    Cocaine when sniffed can lead to ischaemic perforation of the nasal
septum (vasoconstriction due to inhibition of catecholamine uptake).

Cannabis
Taken orally or smoked.
Cannabis = products of *Cannabis sativa*. Two forms:
1. Hashish = resin from flowering tops.
2. Marihuana = chopped leaves and stalk.
Psychic dependence only.

Acute effects
Distorted perception of time, colour, music
Social relaxation
Short term memory is impaired
Hallucinations
Incoordination
Tachycardia
Panic and delirium (bad trip) which may recur after intoxication has
worn off (flashbacks).

Chronic effects
Mild dementia and personality changes — effects disputed.

Opioids
Taken orally, i.v., subcutaneously, smoked.

Several opioids abused — morphine, diamorphine, methadone, pethidine, dipipanone, dextropropoxyphene are commonest. May be taken with other drugs of addiction.

Produce severe physical and psychic dependence with tolerance.

Acute overdose reactions
Pulmonary oedema
Hypoxic reaction — acute respiratory depression (due to irregular
                   potency of street supply or loss of tolerance).
                 — reaction to adulterants or particles in street drug.

Complications of opioid abuse

Infections
Common:
1. hepatitis
2. endocarditis (50% on tricuspid valve; *Staph. aureus* commonest, but also fungal)
3. septicaemia
4. AIDS.
Rare:
Malaria, syphilis, tetanus, osteomyelitis.

Immunological
1. Nephropathy and nephrotic syndrome.
2. Acquired immune deficiency syndrome with *Pneumocystis carinii* pneumonia and Kaposi's sarcoma.
3. False positive serology for syphilis and rheumatoid factor.

Cardiovascular
1. Arrhythmias
2. Emboli.

Pulmonary
1. Ventilation/perfusion defects
2. Embolism by foreign particles
3. Aspiration pneumonia.

Gastrointestinal
1. Constipation
2. Biliary hypertension with raised aminotransferases, alkaline phosphatase and amylase.

Skin
1. Needle tracks, cellulitis and thrombophlebitis
2. Urticaria.

Nervous system
1. Post-anoxic encephalopathy
2. Transverse myelopathy and paraplegia.

Obstetric
1. Low birth weight or prematurity
2. Neonatal withdrawal syndrome (mortality 50%).

Withdrawal syndrome
At~8 h — yawning; sweating; rhinorrhoea; tearing; anxiety.
~20 h — gooseflesh ('cold turkey'); chills; sweating; panic.
~24–48 h — nausea and vomiting; diarrhoea; hypertension; fever.
Up to 1 week — muscle cramps.
Up to several months — insomnia.
Syndrome accompanied by craving for drug.
Syndrome suppressed with methadone (20 mg in divided doses first
3 days then 10 mg for 3 days) or clonidine (experimental).
Syndrome precipitated by opioid antagonists.

Nicotine
Tobacco smoke is a complex mixture which includes nicotine.
Nicotine is an alkaloid in the leaves of *Nicotiana tabacum*.

Actions
1. Stimulates then blocks nicotinic cholinergic receptors (raised blood
   pressure, tachycardia, cutaneous and splanchnic vasoconstriction).
2. Stimulates: vomiting centre, ADH secretion.
3. Stimulation of respiration (carotid body reflex).
4. Cocaine-like stimulatory action on brain due to blockade of amine
   reuptake by neurones.
   Powerfully addicting with psychic and physical elements. Tolerance
occurs. Withdrawal state (constipation, increased appetite, nicotine
craving).
Smokers have *accelerated metabolism* of:
nicotine
imipramine
phenacetin
caffeine
propoxyphene
pentazocine
theophylline.
but *normal metabolism* of:
diazepam
desipramine
pethidine
warfarin
ethanol.

Adverse effects
Strong correlation with:
Ischaemic heart disease
Cancers of lung, trachea, oesophagus, lip, mouth and tongue.
Chronic bronchitis and emphysema, tuberculosis, cor pulmonale.
Aortic aneurysm
Hernia
Peripheral vascular disease
Premature delivery, small babies, raised perinatal mortality.

Possible beneficial effects
Associated with decreased incidence of ulcerative colitis and
Alzheimer's disease.

Treatment
High degree of motivation important.
Some can abruptly stop.
Others can undertake gradual withdrawal or use graded filters (allow
    decreasing amount of smoke inhalation).
Nicotine chewing gum (Nicorette) in 2 mg and 4 mg/piece can be
    prescribed. Nicotine in gum is resin bound so absorption is slower
    than during smoking (and so less satisfying) and depends on speed
    of chewing. Most of the nicotine is absorbed in first 30 minutes:
    chewing one 4 mg piece of gum every hour produces plasma
    nicotine levels similar to those of heavy smokers. Nicorette is used
    to control withdrawal symptoms while behavioural components are
    overcome.
Success rate 15–30% at 1 year.

Solvents
Volatile hydrocarbons — petrol, lighter fuel
                        — glue solvents (toluene, acetone)
                        — paint thinners, hair lacquer
Inhaled from a bag or rag — often a group activity.

Produces
Euphoria and exhilaration (like alcohol) followed by auditory or visual
hallucinations. Then cerebral depression: ataxia, blurred vision,
disorientation, drowsiness.

Adverse effects
Rarely serious in most cases BUT:
occasionally renal damage
toluene encephalopathy sometimes with abdominal pain, nausea and
    vomiting.
asphyxial death.
may produce tolerance and occasional withdrawal symptoms.

22. Legal and practical aspects of prescribing

Medicines Act (1968)
Classifies medicines into three categories:
1. *General sales list preparations*: may be purchased from any shop or even a vending machine.
2. *Pharmacy only medicines*: supplied to a patient by a registered pharmacist without prescription.
3. *Prescription only medicines (POM)*: only supplied by pharmacist on the prescription of registered medical (or dental) practitioner.
   a. provisionally registered doctors cannot write prescriptions for POM for dispensing outside hospital.
   b. provision for supply of small quantities of POM in emergency to patient provided that it has been prescribed previously by a doctor and it is not a controlled drug (see below) or one of a number of other substances such as barbiturates (except for epilepsy).

Misuse of Drugs Act (1971)
This provides control over the misuse of drugs by defining the conditions for the manufacture, supply and possession of certain drugs. These are put into 3 classes:
Class A: Cocaine, morphine and similar opioids. Injections of codeine and similar opioids and of amphetamine.
Class B: Oral amphetamine, barbiturates, cannabis, pentazocine and codeine.
Class C: Buprenorphine, diethylpropion and similar stimulants, most benzodiazepines.

Misuse of Drugs Regulations (1985)
Defines the classes of persons authorised to possess and supply controlled drugs. These regulations divide the drugs into 5 schedules — each with different control regulations:
Schedule 1: Drugs not used medicinally e.g. cannabis and lysergide.
Schedule 2: Diamorphine + similar opioids, amphetamine, cocaine, quinalbarbitone.
Schedule 3: Buprenorphine, pentazocine, diethylpropion.

Schedule 4: Benzodiazepines and pemoline.
Schedule 5: Preparations which because of their strength are practically exempt from Controlled Drug requirements.

Schedules 2 and 3 (appear in the British National Formulary marked CD (controlled drug))
A prescription for a drug in these schedules must conform to the following rules:
1. In the doctor's own handwriting in ink or other indelible medium it must state:
    a. name and address of patient
    b. dose to be taken
    c. form (e.g. tablets, mixture) and, where appropriate, concentration of the drug
    d. total quantity of preparation to be supplied
    e. quantities and concentrations written in figures and words
    f. doctor's signature and date
    g. repeat prescriptions are not permitted, but the prescription can instruct the pharmacist to dispense in instalments.
2. The doctor's address need not be written but must appear on the prescription.
In addition:
3. The prescriber's address must be within the UK
4. The prescription must be presented within 13 weeks of the date on the prescription
5. The pharmacist must be assured of the genuineness of the signature before dispensing.

   Doctors have a general right to possess these drugs and to administer and prescribe them subject to:
1. The keeping of a register of prescription and stocks of these drugs (usually done for the doctor by the nurses or pharmacist in hospital or retail practice). Entries must be indelible and chronological. Alterations must be accompanied by an explanation.
2. The keeping of such drugs in a locked receptacle (not a locked car or case).
   Patients may possess such drugs only if perscribed. It is an offence to fail to disclose to a prescribing doctor that another doctor has already prescribed a controlled drug.
   It is an offence for a doctor to issue an incomplete prescription, and for a pharmacist to dispense a controlled drug unless all the information required by law is given in the prescription.

Notification and Supply to Addicts Regulations (1973)
1. Doctors are *obliged* to notify (within 7 days) to the Chief Medical Officer at the Home Office the name, sex, date of birth, address,

date of attendance, and NHS number of any patient suspected of addiction to: cocaine, dextromoramide, diamorphine, dipipanone, hydrocodone, hydromorphone, levorphanol, methadone, morphine, opium, oxycodone, pethidine, phenazocine and piritramide.
2. Failure to notify is an offence and can result in withdrawal of the right to prescribe controlled drugs.
3. Except for treatment of organic disease and injury, doctors are not allowed to prescribe controlled drugs to addicts unless they have a licence from the Secretary of State to do so. Thus prescription to addicts is limited to doctors specialised in their management.

Practical aspects of prescribing.
1. Write legibly with particular care to specification of dose (watch the decimal points, avoid confusing mg and µg, etc).
2. Clearly indicate the drug.
3. Specify full name, address and age of patient.
4. Specify precisely the strength of mixtures, creams, tablets.
5. Give clear instructions as to dose frequency, duration of treatment, and/or total amount to be supplied.
   Give dosage >1 gram as fractions of gram, e.g. 1.5 g
   <1 gram as milligrams, e.g. 500 mg, not 0.5 g
   <1 mg as micrograms, e.g. 100 micrograms not 0.1 mg.
   Where decimals are unavoidable, a zero should be written before the decimal point.
   Liquid medicines are usually prescribed in multiples of 10 doses of 10 ml, the adult dose, i.e. 50, 100, 150, 200, 300 or 500 ml.
   Topical liquid preparations: — 500 ml suitable for whole body
   — 200 ml for limbs
   — 100 ml for small areas, e.g. face.
   Eye and ear drops usually ordered in volumes of 10 ml; inhalations and sprays as 25 ml; eye lotions, gargles and mouth washes as 200 ml.
   Creams and ointments usually determined by the size of manufacturer's pack. As guide, whole body requires 100–200 g; medium areas 25–50 g; and small areas 5–25 g.
6. Do not leave large spaces which allow alteration or addition to your prescription.
7. Sign and date the prescription. Add your name and address. A telephone number is also helpful.
8. If in doubt, look it up or ask.
9. Unless otherwise specified, the name of the drug will automatically be written on the label by the pharmacist.
   Best to use simple English words and arabic numerals in writing prescriptions. Some Latin abbreviations are commonly used (not advised) by some prescribers:

a.c., ante cibum	before food
b.d., bis in die	twice a day (b.i.d. is also used)
o.d., omni die	every day
o.m., omni mane	every morning
o.n., omni nocte	every night
p.c., post cibum	after food
p.o., per os	by mouth
p.r.n., pro re nata	as required
q.d.s., quater in die	four times a day (q.i.d. also used)
q.s., quantum sufficiat	a sufficiency, enough
rep., repetatur	let it be repeated
s.o.s., si opus sit	if necessary. Confine s.o.s. to prescriptions to be repeated once only and to use p.r.n. where many repetitions are intended.
stat., statim	immediately
t.d.s., ter in die	three times a day (t.i.d. also used)

Compliance with therapy
If after accurate diagnosis and appropriate prescribing the patient fails to take the drug the whole exercise is futile. Patients who fail to take therapy are called *non-compliers*.

Incidence
Much greater than expected or realised.
Always suspect non-compliance if treatment fails.
20% patients in general practice may not take their prescription for dispensing.
33% patients are non-compliers.
33% patients are poor compliers.
   Many determinants of compliance described but impossible to identify such individuals accurately.
   Patients may comply with one regimen but not another.
   Non-compliance more likely when:
1. Patients are very young or very old or psychiatrically ill.
2. Treatment is chronic.
3. No obvious connection between treatment and subjectively perceived benefit.
4. Failure to understand nature or importance of illness, side effects, and/or treatment.
5. Complex treatment — too many drugs or too frequent administration.
   Non-compliance may reflect failure of doctor to identify main reason for patient's visit: many patients do not always expect a prescription.

Diagnosis
Difficult in clinical practice. Can be done by:
1. Relaxed and friendly doctor-patient relationship may allow patient to discuss compliance.
2. Comparison of amount of drug left with expected consumption.
3. Assessment of clinical effect.
4. Plasma, urine or salivary drug level monitoring.

Treatment
Few trials to investigate effects of these measures. Probably important are:
1. Clear instructions about treatment, disease, etc. Write it down for patient if necessary.
2. Simple drug regime: twice daily regime known to be better than three or four times a day; reduce number of separate drug prescriptions (use combination tablets if appropriate).
3. In certain cases, e.g. schizophrenia, intramuscular depot injections can be used.
4. Regular follow-up and evaluation of patient response.
   If a drug is necessary, then so is compliance, and it is worth spending time to obtain it.

Index

Page numbers in *italics* refer to figures and tables